Delmar's Medical Transcription Handbook

Second Edition

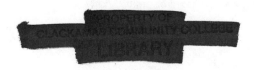

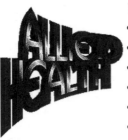

Delmar's Medical Transcription Handbook

Second Edition

Rachelle S. Blake, M.A., R. M. T.

Transcription Manager, The Polyclinic, Seattle, Washington
Chief Executive Officer, Alphascribe, Inc., Denver, Colorado/Seattle, Washington
Founder, The Transcription Institute and International Medical Transcriptionists
    Association, Denver, Colorado and Seattle, Washington

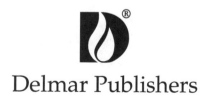

Delmar Publishers

an International Thomson Publishing company I(T)P

Albany • Bonn • Boston • Cincinnati • Detroit • London • Madrid
Melbourne • Mexico City • New York • Pacific Grove • Paris • San Francisco
Singapore • Tokyo • Toronto • Washington

Cover Design: Scott Keidong

Delmar Staff

Publisher: Susan Simpfenderfer
Acquisitions Editor: Marlene Pratt
Developmental Editor: Jill Rembetski
Project Editor: William Trudell

Production Coordinator: James Zayicek
Art and Design Coordinator: Timothy J. Conners
Marketing Manager: Darryl L. Caron

COPYRIGHT © 1998
Delmar is a division of Thomson Learning. The Thomson Learning logo is a registered trademark used herein under license.

Printed in the United States of America
4 5 6 7 8 9 10 XXX 03 02 01 00

For more information, contact Delmar, 3 Columbia Circle, PO Box 15015, Albany, NY 12212-0515; or find us on the World Wide Web at http://www.delmar.com

International Division List

Japan:
Thomson Learning
Palaceside Building 5F
1-1-1 Hitotsubashi, Chiyoda-ku
Tokyo 100 0003 Japan
Tel: 813 5218 6544
Fax: 813 5218 6551

Australia/New Zealand
Nelson/Thomson Learning
102 Dodds Street
South Melbourne, Victoria 3205
Australia
Tel: 61 39 685 4111
Fax: 61 39 685 4199

UK/Europe/Middle East:
Thomson Learning
Berkshire House
168-173 High Holborn
London
WC1V 7AA United Kingdom
Tel: 44 171 497 1422
Fax: 44 171 497 1426

Latin America:
Thomson Learning
Seneca, 53
Colonia Polanco
11560 Mexico D.F. Mexico
Tel: 525-281-2906
Fax: 525-281-2656

Canada:
Nelson/Thomson Learning
1120 Birchmount Road
Scarborough, Ontario
Canada M1K 5G4
Tel: 416-752-9100
Fax: 416-752-8102

Asia:
Thomson Learning
60 Albert Street, #15-01
Albert Complex
Singapore 189969
Tel: 65 336 6411
Fax: 65 336 7411

Library of Congress Cataloging-in-Publication Data:
Blake, Rachelle S., 1964–
    Delmar's medical transcription handbook / Rachelle S. Blake.
—2nd ed.
      p.   cm.
    Rev. ed. of: The medical transcriptionist's handbook / Rachelle S. Blake. c1993.
    Includes bibliographical references and index.
    ISBN 0-8273-8325-8 (alk. paper)
    1. Medical transcription—Handbooks, manuals, etc. I. Blake, Rachelle S., 1964– Medical Transcriptionist's handbook.
II. Title.
    [DNLM: 1. Medical Records—handbooks. 2. Medical Secretaries—handbooks. W 39 B636d 1998]
R728.8.B54   1988
653'.18—dc21
DNLM/DLC
for Library of Congress

97-18408
CIP

Contents

Appendices 211

Preface

Direction and Objective: *Delmar's Medical Transcription Handbook,* Second Edition, is directed to students of medical transcription as well as to currently practicing medical transcriptionists who work in hospitals, clinics and physician's offices, for professional medical transcription services, and as independent contractors. The objective of this handbook is to provide medical transcriptionists with:

- a compilation of comprehensive answers to common questions and problems encountered when transcribing medical dictation
- a medical perspective regarding the documentation of records
- a source of basic information and guidelines for style, grammar and specific medical transcription mechanics
- a fundamental training manual, including a separate workbook with practical exercises for the medical transcription student
- a practical supplement to the medical transcriptionist's personal library of medical texts and style guides, word books, dictionaries and grammar texts

Features: *Delmar's Medical Transcription Handbook,* Second Edition, features a chapter-by-chapter breakdown of medical transcription mechanics such as abbreviations, numbers, plural and possessive forms, and capitalization. The handbook includes general guidelines, examples and applications for basic medical transcription as well as in-depth coverage of editing and spelling techniques and techniques for formatting medical records. New to this edition are comprehensive key words for each chapter, indicated in bold print. The user of this text should be able to define these words upon the completion of each chapter. Additionally, the key words may be used as study aids. Also new to this edition are chapters that detail the business and marketing aspects of medical transcription. The text includes a number of appendices that provide the medical transcriptionist with specialized information about common medical terms and abbreviations, Greek and Latin medical words, units of measure and laboratory data, as well as a comprehensive reference guide to medical transcription resources.

Although other training manuals and reference texts in medical transcription exist, *Delmar's Medical Transcription Handbook,* Second Edition, is unique because it serves as both a reference manual and a textbook. Future transcriptionists can use the text in their studies, then continue to use the book in their daily work as medical transcriptionists. Practicing medical transcriptionists can use the book as a handy reference guide.

Organization: Each chapter in *Delmar's Medical Transcription Handbook,* Second Edition, begins with an overview, or summary, of the chapter's particular focus and its associated key terms. Further, each chapter contains detailed explanations and specific examples of concepts introduced. Finally, each chapter includes a summary of concepts, providing a recap of the major topics discussed.

New to the second edition is the *Workbook to Accompany Delmar's Medical Transcription Handbook,* which supplements this text. The workbook provides a study aid that will enhance the medical transcription student's absorption of the topics covered in each chapter in the textbook. It also includes review and revision activities for each chapter, key word exercises and optional appendices exercises, as well as practice tests for each chapter to ensure proper preparation for closed-book, in-class examinations. Also new in this edition are additional exercises such as word find, crossword puzzles and scrambled words, which provide helpful study aids and concept-retention mechanisms.

Instructor's Supplements: The accompanying instructor's manual to *Delmar's Medical Transcription Handbook,* Second Edition, includes an overview of each part presented in the handbook and the criterion performance objectives the student should achieve for each chapter. The manual also contains solutions to workbook exercises, activities, and practice tests, impromptu, informal quiz suggestions for each chapter, and supplementary objective tests consisting of multiple-choice, short answer, and matching questions, with corresponding test answers. These supplementary objective tests are appropriate to use as closed-book, in-class examinations.

About the Author: Rachelle Blake, author of *Delmar's Medical Transcription Handbook,* has worked in the legal and medical transcription industry for more than 15 years. Her vocational experience includes working as a medical office clerk, a medical transcriptionist, a medical office administrator, a medical transcription supervisor, a medical transcription service operations manager, an instructor in medical transcription, a medical transcription manager, and a chief executive officer for a major metropolitan medical, legal and broadcast transcription service. Blake attended Boulder College and the University of Denver, with a master's degree in medical office administration. She has served several internships and apprenticeships and has been trained and employed in hospitals, clinics and physicians' offices nationwide. She has taught at Denver Technical College and Colorado Free University, both in Denver, Colorado. She is the founder and executive director of The Transcription Institute, which offers, among other educational opportunities, a correspondence course in medical transcription. Blake is also the founder and executive director of the International Medical Transcriptionists Association (IMTA), a professional organization for medical transcriptionists. She has served as the chief executive officer of Alphascribe, Inc., a medical, legal and broadcast medical transcription service, for the past nine years. She administrated for nine years the contract medical transcription services for Aurora Associates of Otolaryngology, Aurora, Colorado. She is currently the medical transcription manager for The Polyclinic, a 90-staff physician multispecialty clinic located in Seattle, Washington, with over 20 in-house and home-based transcriptionists.

Acknowledgments: I would like to thank the following persons for the inspiration, help, advice and support they have provided throughout my career as a medical transcriptionist, a medical transcription service manager/owner, and an instructor and author. I also gratefully acknowledge those whom I have inadvertently failed to mention, who aided in the creation of this book. Without these individuals, this project would not have been possible.

My family, including my husband Richard Roy Blake, without whose love and assurance this work could not have been created and renewed; my lovely and talented daughters Ashleigh Annette and Angelique Rachelle Robin; my beloved son Jean-Richard, my mother Lettie Annette Scott, and my grandmother Bessie Craddock, who provided me with inspiration and sustenance throughout their too-short lives; my father John Scott Sr.; my "second" parents Floyd and Connie Blake; my aunts Leatha Bailey and Ruth Lynch; my uncle J. Richard Peck; my brothers John A. Scott, II, and Kai A. I. Scott; my dear friend and "sister" Robin Brantford Anderson; my lifelong friend Cassandra Jue-Low; my most rewarding student, and often profound teacher in life, Sue Felton; Debbie and Jerry Hanlon; Debbie Prodoehl; Lora Moynihan; and a host of other students, friends and family members who have given me their undying support.

Those who inspired and assisted me in the development of this book include: Betty Schechter; Inell Bolls-Gaither; Susan Brodie; the Students of Denver Technical College, 1989–90; the students of Colorado Free University, 1993–94; H. Patrick Carr, M.D.; Linda Houlihan; Irene Hughes; the late Rick W. Rasband, M.D.; Steven O'Brien, M.D. and Debra Ganter, M.D., two supportive former medical residents who helped give me somatic strength; Diane Schauger; Jennifer Martin; Donna Avila-Weil; and Arlene Atchison Stolte.

The author would also like to thank the following reviewers:

Bonnie J. Lindsey
Arkansas State University,
Mountain Home Campus
Mountain Home, AR

Brenda A. Potter, Instructor
Medical Secretary Program
NW Technical College
Fargo, ND

Jeannette Gaynor
Southern Ohio College, Northeast
Akron, OH

Betsy Murren
Beta Training Service
Swarthmore, PA

Darlene Walker, Instructor
Learning Tree University
Sylmar, CA

Michelle Johnson
New Ulm Medical Center
New Ulm, MN

Susan D. Steinriede, Ph.D.
Trident Technical College
Charleston, SC

Part One

Introduction to Medical Transcription

Chapter 1

What Is Medical Transcription?

Overview: Welcome to the exciting and challenging career of medical transcription. The author hopes that you will find this handbook helpful in performing your duties as a medical transcriptionist and that this handbook will save you a great deal of time when searching for the proper word, format or method to use when transcribing. Before we dive into the great wealth of mechanics the medical transcriptionist uses, however, let us first ask ourselves: *What is medical transcription, and what do medical transcriptionists do?*

Key Words

AAMT

allied health professional team

anatomy and physiology

chain of command

clerk

confidential

dictation

discipline

document

editing

ergonomics

hand-eye coordination

health information team

Hippocratic Oath

independent contractor

keyboarding/word processing

language mechanisms

medical records

medical records supervisor

medical terminology

medical transcription

medical transcription service

medical transcriptionist

medicine

mental deciphering

pathophysiology

pharmacology

proofer

self-commitment

speech idiosyncracies

subpoenaed

transcribe

word breakdowns

work environment

1–A A Brief History of the Documentation of Medicine

Medicine, the preservation of health, the prevention of illness and the treatment of disease processes, is one of the most basic elements of life. With its earliest foundations based in religion, medicine was first practiced thousands of years ago in the Stone Age. Unfortunately, Neanderthal man did not have a written alphabet, so he was unable to leave a record of his medical concepts and philosophy.

Later, medicine was practiced by medicine men, or "shamans." To early Native Americans, medicine included anything having a religious or therapeutic orientation, from objects such as bows, arrowheads or stones, to injuries such as a lacerated arm, a bruised leg or a wounded knee. These medicine men practiced or "made" medicine, either through ceremonies or natural herbs and preparations. Unfortunately, however, the techniques they used were still not easily passed on; documentation, in the form of petroglyphs or picture-writing on rocks, was crude and limited, and simple pictorial representations of treatments often were confusing or misunderstood.

A more advanced documentation of medicine was accomplished during the fourth and fifth centuries B.C. It is generally accepted that the art of practicing medicine as a documented scientific method was begun by the Greek physician Hippocrates in about 500 B.C. Hippocrates authored a collection of works known as the Hippocratic Corpus, which includes the **Hippocratic Oath** (Figure 1–1), which physicians take upon their entrance into the field. (Some medical schools use statements and prayers at graduation ceremonies, such as the Declaration of Geneva or the Prayer of Maimonides. A medical dictionary can be consulted for the specific text of each of these.)

HIPPOCRATIC OATH

"I swear by Apollo the physician, and Aesculapius, and Hygeia, and Panacea, and all the gods and goddesses, that according to my ability and judgment, I will keep this oath and its stipulation—to reckon him who taught me this art equally dear to me as my parents, to share my substance with him, and to relieve his necessities if required; to look upon his offspring in the same footing as my own brothers, and to teach them this art if they shall wish to learn it, without fee or stipulation, and that by precept, lecture, and every other mode of instruction, I will impart a knowledge of the art to my own sons, and those of my teachers, and to disciples bound by a stipulation and oath according to the law of medicine, but to none other.

"I will follow that system of regimen which, according to my ability and judgment, I consider for the benefit of my patients, and abstain from whatever is deleterious and mischievous. I will give no deadly medicine to anyone if asked, nor suggest any such counsel, and in like manner I will not give to a woman a pessary to produce

---

Figure 1–1   The Hippocratic Oath

abortion. With purity and with holiness I will pass my life and practice my art. I will not cut persons laboring under the stone, but will leave this to be done by men who are practitioners of this work. Into whatever houses I enter, I will go into them for the benefit of the sick, and I will abstain from every voluntary act of mischief and corruption; and, further, from the seduction of females or males, of freeman and slaves. Whatever, in connection with my professional practice, or not in connection with it, I see or hear, in the life of men, which ought not to be spoken of abroad, I will not divulge, as reckoning that all such should be kept secret.

"While I continue to keep this Oath unviolated, may it be granted to me to enjoy life and the practice of this art, respected by all men, in all times. But should I trespass and violate this Oath, may the reverse be my lot."

Figure 1–1 continued

As you can see, the documentation and recording of medical procedure and theory are essential links in the long chain of the history of the practice of medicine. You as a medical transcriptionist continue the chain by documenting the art and the process of medicine.

1–B The Medical Transcription Process

What Is Medical Transcription? **Medical transcription** is the act of taking written or dictated medical information and producing a permanent, uniform and legible record of that information in keyboarded form (via a word processor, personal computer, or, increasingly less frequently, a typewriter). To **transcribe** is literally "to change into writing." More traditionally speaking, transcribing is changing oral **dictation** (words spoken, or dictated, for the purpose of writing them down) into written form. The medical information a medical transcriptionist transcribes can vary from office notes regarding a patient's visit to the physician to a specific hospital report such as a pathology or radiology report to a manuscript for publication regarding medical or scientific topics. The information in all cases is considered confidential and should always be treated with sensitivity, privacy and respect. (Review the Hippocratic Oath in Figure 1–1.)

Records describing an encounter between a health care provider and a patient, called **medical records,** are documents governed by laws and scrutinized by members of the legal community. Oftentimes, substantiation of a medical legal claim, an injury involving the law, or medical malpractice hinges upon documentation of the patient's circumstances through her or his medical record. Therefore, medical records have the potential to be **subpoenaed** (ordered to be produced in a court of law) and should be regarded at all times as formal legal documentation. A written note in a patient's chart, a letter of thanks to a referring physician or law office, or a phone conversation to a pharmacist concerning a patient's medication can all be documented, and therefore become part of the patient's official medical record. Further, medical transcription, as part of the medical record, can be used by insurance companies, legal and government entities, and others to compile information about a patient or an individual; thus all documentation related to a patient having sought health care services should be kept undisclosed and private, or **confidential,** at all times. (Confidentiality will be discussed in further detail in subsequent chapters.) Also keep in mind that medical transcription, once complete, should always be orderly, tidy and professional in appearance.

What Is a Medical Transcriptionist? A **medical transcriptionist** is a person who transcribes oral and/or written medical dictation, producing permanent and uniform medical records and information. (See Figure 1–2.) Medical transcriptionists are an integral part of the **allied health professional team**—the nurses, office managers and staff, physicians' assistants and medical assistants, and others whose primary task is to work with the physician in providing medical care. Medical transcriptionists are part secretary, part translator, part editor and part medical assistant; they also must be language specialists. Medical transcriptionists also are key members of the **health information team**—clerks, secretaries, technicians, transcriptionists, medical librarians and other medical personnel—who collect, process, sort, store and retrieve medical information and health care data.

A medical transcriptionist can work in a hospital, at a medical office or clinic or as an **independent contractor** (one who is self-employed with a contractual agreement to perform specific tasks) for a **medical transcription service,** a company that provides medical transcription services for an unassociated and independent facility or client. Transcription duties may be provided at home or at the service, or a transcriptionist may work independently.

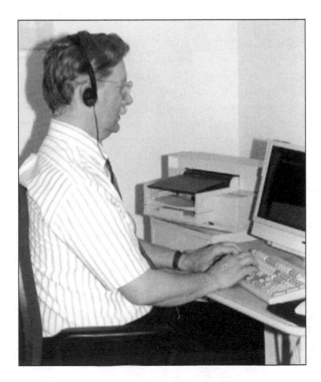

Figure 1–2 A medical transcriptionist at work

Medical transcriptionists many times need to work independently, or with minimal supervision. Therefore, **discipline** (control over one's behavior) and **self-commitment** (pledging to achieve one's goals) are important requirements for becoming a successful medical transcriptionist. Medical transcriptionists must develop skills in listening, **mental deciphering** (figuring out complex concepts or terms in the mind without having to write them down), **hand-eye coordination** (having the hand and eye work in conjunction without focusing on either) and concentration. They also must be able to perform in a high-pressure work environment where there is a specific time in which the transcription task must be completed. Additionally, they must be prepared to deal with a variety of **speech idiosyncracies,** including regional dialects, accents, colloquialisms, foreign language variations and speech impediments. Medical transcriptionists must be familiar with the **ergonomics** of transcription, the science of tailoring the transcription process to the transcriptionist's own anatomical, physiologic and psychological characteristics, in a manner that will blend efficiency with well-being. Ergonomics associated with medical transcription include: being physically and mentally prepared for the work at hand; being familiar with specialized tools that can aid in the transcription of work (such as specially designed keyboards, screen glare guards, etc.); being aware of physical and mental strengths and weaknesses that can be helpful or detrimental; being knowledgeable of hand, back and other bodily exercises to minimize and prevent workplace injury and exhaustion; and having in place support systems (such as groups like the American Association for Medical Transcription, or **AAMT,** and colleagues, close friends and confidants) so feelings can be shared and feedback can be received regarding job stress, personal and professional accomplishments, advancement, and other general, nonconfidential topics associated with work or the workplace.

All medical transcriptionists must be well trained in a variety of disciplines: grammar (the study of words and their roles in a sentence); **keyboarding/word processing** (saving text in computerized form in an internal memory bank or on a magnetized diskette or cassette tape instead of on a piece of paper); **medical terminology** (words specifically related to the medical field); **anatomy and physiology** (the study of the structure and function of the body and its systems); **pathophysiology** (the study of how body functions are affected by disease); and **pharmacology** (the study of drugs and medicines and their effects on living things). Transcriptionists must be able to produce legible, logical and comprehensible reports from oral or written documents that were previously lacking in one or all of these qualities.

Learning to transcribe medical dictation is not extremely difficult, yet it is challenging, therefore, consistent study, self-motivation, continuing education and true dedication are all important requisites.

What Knowledge Is Necessary Regarding Words and How To Use Them? An exhaustive knowledge of words and how to use them are necessary skills for becoming a successful medical transcriptionist. A transcriptionist must be fluent in different forms of **word breakdowns,** such as phonemics (keys to pronunciation), etymology (study of word origins), phraseology (the study of sentences and phrases), as well as in the use of acronyms (words that are made from the first letter of a group of words) homonyms (words that are spelled alike and pronounced alike, but are different in meaning), synonyms (words with similar meanings) and antonyms *(words* with opposite meanings).

What Does a Medical Transcriptionist Have To Know About Editing? **Editing** (assembling or reassembling a word, group of words or **document**—one or more pages of text—by cutting, pasting, adding, deleting and rearranging) is another important component to medical transcription. A medical transcriptionist has to know when, as well as how, to edit. Some of the **language mechanisms** she or he must use in editing include using correct words, grammar, punctuation, numbers, abbreviations, plurals, possessives, compound words, pronouns and contractions.

A medical transcriptionist must know when to edit (when it would not affect the dictator's meaning or style) and how to edit (how to transform the transcription into clear, concise and more logical expressions of the same information).

1-C The Medical Transcription Environment

It is important to understand the **work environment** in which a medical transcriptionist performs his or her duties, because many factors in transcribing and editing a physician's dictation depend on the physical proximity of the dictator to the transcriptionist. If the physician can be easily contacted for questions and/or revisions, the transcriptionist may be able to transcribe more liberally. However, if the physician can only be contacted through a series of steps in a **chain of command,** then the transcriptionist must be more rigid and rule-adhering when transcribing the dictation.

As previously mentioned, medical transcriptionists work in hospitals, clinics and medical offices, for outside medical transcription services, and in their own homes, either as independent contractors for other services or for services they independently own and operate. The chain of command is different for each of these settings. Therefore, medical transcriptionists should be aware of each and of the proximity of the transcriptionist to the physician to determine how readily the physician will be able to make changes to and/or critiques of the dictation. After the medical transcriptionist is aware of the chain of command, he or she will know how much or how little flexibility there will be when editing the dictation, as well as how much interaction will be needed with the physician to become familiar with her or his style. Keep in mind that the organization of each facility can vary from location to location; the flowcharts that follow illustrate only one example of the chain of command that may exist at the facility in which the medical transcriptionist works.

Figure 1–3 illustrates the medical transcription work environment of a hospital.

In the hospital setting, the medical transcriptionist typically has little direct contact with the dictating physician. The normal route of progress from dictation to transcription may be as follows: The physician dictates a report, indicates to the medical staff office that the dictation has been made, and places it in a receptacle designated for medical transcription in the medical records department. The transcriptionist takes the dictation, transcribes it, prints it out if necessary and places it in a location designated for completed reports. The report is then either charted to await the physician's perusal and signature, or it is placed in a designated area for

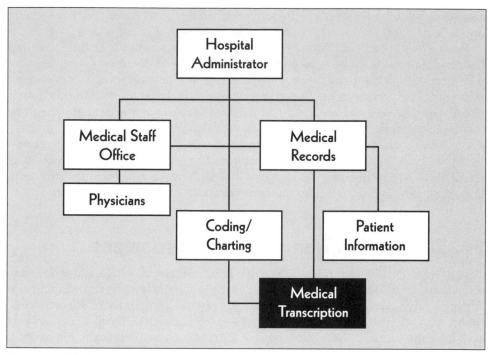

Figure 1–3   The hospital as a medical transcription work environment

completed medical transcription. Therefore, contact with the physician may be limited. In the majority of instances, the physician and the transcriptionist do not make any direct contact, but rely on the medical records department as an intermediary.

Figure 1–4 illustrates the medical transcription work environment of a medical office.

In the medical office, the medical transcriptionist may have quite a bit of direct contact with the dictating physician. Sometimes the medical office administrator may act as an intermediary, conveying messages from the transcriptionist to the physician, or the transcriptionist may go directly to the physician with questions or problems. The normal route of progress from dictation to transcription may be as follows: The physician dictates a report and delivers it either to the medical office administrator or directly to the transcriptionist. The transcriptionist takes the dictation, transcribes it, prints it out if necessary, and gives it either to the physician to be signed or to the medical office administrator for initial clearance.

Figure 1–5 illustrates the medical transcription work environment of an outside-the-home medical transcription service.

In an outside-the-home medical transcription service, the medical transcriptionist usually has no direct contact with the dictating physician. The normal route of progress from dictation to transcription may be as follows: The physician dictates a report and delivers it either to the medical office administrator or **medical records supervisor** (a staff member who supervises the work and personnel of a medical records department) or directly to the medical transcription supervisor at

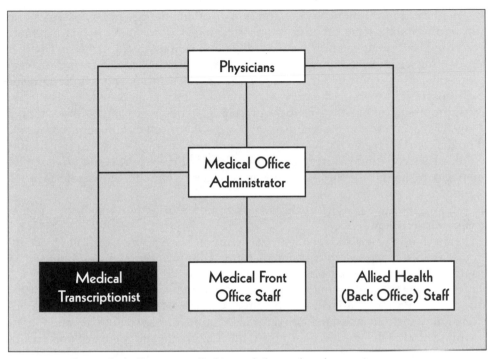

Figure 1–4 The medical office as a medical transcription work environment

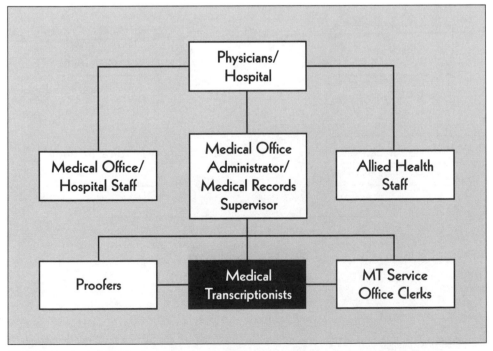

Figure 1–5 An outside-the-home medical transcription service as a medical transcription work environment

the medical transcription service. The transcriptionist either physically picks up (on audiocassette tapes) the dictation or remotely downloads it (via a remote recording or digital dictation system, which will be explained further in Chapter 2). The transcriptionist then takes the dictation, transcribes it, and gives the saved, word-processed report to either the **proofer,** an allied technician who proofreads the transcribed report (in the previous two instances, the medical transcriptionist must proofread his or her own work), or a **clerk,** an office assistant with secretarial as well as reception and other duties, who will either print out the report or resave it on disk and then give the work to the supervisor. After the supervisor's critique, either a disk containing the report or a hard copy of the report is sent to the office manager or medical records supervisor, or directly back to the physician to be signed.

Figure 1–6 illustrates the medical transcription work environment of a home-based transcription service.

In the home-based independent transcription service, the medical transcriptionist works independently at home and usually has minimal or limited direct contact with the dictating physician. The home-based transcriptionist may be a subcontractor for another medical transcription service, or he or she may contract directly with a medical facility or health care provider. A home-based transcriptionist may pick up tapes and deliver transcription, or use remote dictation, transcription and delivery mechanisms. With a pick-up and delivery method of

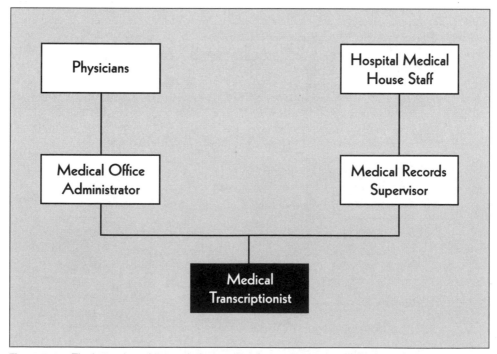

Figure 1–6   The home-based transcription service as a medical transcription work environment

transcription, the route of progress from dictation to transcription may proceed in the following fashion: The physician or hospital medical staff dictates a report and delivers it either to the medical office administrator, medical clinic or office staff, or a hospital's medical records supervisor. The home-based medical transcriptionist, in turn, picks up the dictation from the medical office or medical records department. The transcriptionist then takes the dictation, transcribes it, and returns it to the medical office administrator or hospital medical records supervisor. After a possible critique by the medical office administrator or hospital medical records supervisor, the report goes back to the physician to be signed. The physician, on occasion, may personally interact with the medical transcriptionist.

Summary of Concepts

- The documentation and recording of medical procedure and theory have been essential to the practice of medicine throughout history.
- Medical transcription is the act of producing a permanent, uniform and legible record of medical information in keyboarded form.
- Medical records are regarded as formal legal documentation and should be kept confidential and professional-appearing at all times.
- A medical transcriptionist, a person who transcribes oral and/or written dictation, is an integral part of the allied health professional team, being part secretary, part translator, part editor and part medical assistant.
- A medical transcriptionist must be disciplined and committed, as well as possess mental deciphering and hand-eye coordination skills. A medical transcriptionist must be able to recognize speech idiosyncracies and must be well versed in grammar, keyboarding/word processing, medical terminology, word breakdowns, editing and language mechanisms.
- To get a better feel for the chain of command that a medical transcriptionist must follow, he or she must be familiar with the four major medical transcription work environments—the hospital, medical office, medical transcription service and home-based transcription service.

Chapter 2

Medical Transcription Transcribing Tools

Overview: The greatest tool medical transcriptionists have at their fingertips is their collective intelligence—the knowledge gained over the many hours spent honing their skills. However, medical transcriptionists also use other important tools—various types of equipment and reference materials—in their trade. Some basic equipment a medical transcriptionist may have at his or her workstation, or the area in which the transcriptionist works, would minimally include the following: a transcriber, a computer with word processing software, and a printer or typewriter. Transcribers, originally simple machines that played audiocassette tapes, have evolved into complex mechanisms such as computerized voice processing machines, voice synthesizers and remote digital dictation systems. These recent dictation and transcription innovations, and how they are helping to transform the medical transcription field into one of the fastest-growing allied health careers is discussed next.

Key Words

analog system

audiocassette voice transcriber

binary code

centralization

cue

dictator

digital signals

digital system

digital voice processing

microcassette transcriber

mini-cassette transcriber

remote dictation

remote transcription

review

standard transcriber

transcriber

transcript

transcription ports

voice synthesizer

2–A Traditional Dedicated Transcribers

The transcriber is essential to the medical transcriptionist. A **transcriber** is a machine that allows the transcriptionist to take oral dictation, decipher and encode it, and turn the spoken words into written material. The transcriber is the device that makes it possible to transform the voice recordings of a **dictator** (a physician or other medical professional who dictates medical information) into a **transcript** (printed document).

Parts of the Transcriber

The traditional dedicated (or self-contained, independently functioning) **audio-cassette voice transcriber** consists of a control base (where the cassette is inserted and controls are located), headphones and a foot pedal. The transcriber usually has speed, tone and volume controls. Each transcriptionist can adjust these controls to suit his or her needs. For example, a beginning transcriptionist will frequently turn the speed to a low setting, so the dictation can be heard at a slower rate than the actual manner in which the physician dictated. If the dictator's speech has a nasal tonality or stuttering style, a change in the tone control may be necessary. Volume may also need to be controlled from dictator to dictator, as some physicians speak quite loudly, while others are difficult to hear. (See the microcassette transcriber in Figure 2–1.)

As with most audiocassette players, there are also play, stop, rewind and fast forward buttons on the base control board. These controls are useful to **cue**

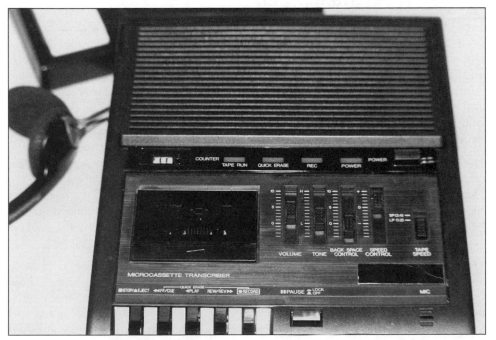

Figure 2–1 A microcassette transcriber

(preview by fast-forwarding) or **review** (scan by rewinding) tapes that have not yet been transcribed, or when the foot pedals are lacking any of these controls. However, the foot pedal is primarily used for playing and rewinding the dictation.

In most cases, the play pedal is on the right side or in the center; however, sometimes it is on the left side. There usually is a rewind pedal, either on the right or left side. The fast forward pedal can be either on the foot pedal on the right, left, top or center, or, less frequently, on the base. Sometimes there is a footrest in the center section. Check the directions for use before beginning to transcribe. Many newer transcribers contain an automatic backspace function, which allows the transcriber to review a small amount of dictation automatically after stopping the play function. This feature is very helpful for medical transcriptionists, as it makes it easier for them to maintain typing speed without having to stop to rewind. A secondary benefit is that there is less wear and tear on the foot pedal, because the rewind pedal is used to a lesser extent.

Most foot pedals are used in the following manner: Push the right side of the foot pedal to play and the left side to rewind; take your foot off the pedal to stop it from playing temporarily as you transcribe; always listen to an earful or play just a few words more than you can transcribe, so you can continue keying as you take your foot off the play pedal; press the play pedal to continue hearing the dictation. The goal with using the audiocassette transcriber is hand-foot/eye-ear coordination—having the hands, feet, eyes and ears all working together to achieve the process of transcribing.

2–B Types of Transcribers

The Standard Audiocassette Transcriber   The **standard transcriber** uses standard audio tapes ($3^{15}/_{16}'' \times 2^{1}/_{2}''$), historically the most commonly used type of tape in the general marketplace. These cassettes are often used in commercial audio recordings and with most types of portable and stereo cassette recorders and players. Some medical transcription environments, such as hospitals, clinics and medical transcription services, continue to use these models. The cassettes are sold everywhere, from supermarkets and department stores to music specialty stores.

The Microcassette Transcriber   The **microcassette transcriber** utilizes the smallest cassette tape on the market today, the micro-sized audiocassette tape ($2'' \times 1^{1}/_{4}''$). Microcassettes are utilized by physicians' offices, clinics, and hospitals because of their easy use and because the dictating machines that accommodate them are handheld, pocket-sized models. The actual cassettes are also usually sold in supermarkets and department stores, as well as in business supply stores.

The Mini-Cassette Transcriber   The **mini-cassette transcriber** employs a cassette tape size whose use is almost exclusively limited to transcribing machines. These mini-sized audio tapes are $2^{3}/_{16}'' \times 1^{3}/_{8}''$, only slightly larger than the microcassette, but microcassette transcribers usually cannot accommodate mini-cassettes and vice versa. Mini-cassettes are frequently used by physicians who have established practices, as they preceded microcassettes, and many physicians still continue to use and treasure their somewhat out-of-date mini-cassette dictating machines. Mini-cassettes generally are only sold in dictating specialty stores.

2–C Other Transcribing Tools

Although most transcriptionists will ultimately have at least some and possibly the majority of their experience working with an audiocassette transcriber, these devices are being replaced by other transcribing tools in large hospitals, large medical transcription services and other medical transcription work environments. Some of these devices will be discussed next.

Computerized Digital Voice Processing Machines

Digital voice processing machines are computer-based transcribing units. The dictator's voice is digitized, or recorded and encoded, into a specialized computer, which converts the voice into a **binary code** (a computer mathematical code using 0s and 1s). These codes, or **digital signals,** are then saved to the hard disk drive of the computer.

An audiocassette transcriber uses an **analog system** instead of a **digital system.** An analog system uses a direct measurement of the quality and quantity of the voice being recorded, and the voice is recorded and played back much like the way it was dictated; a digital system uses a method of converting the voice into digits and then decoding the digits back into actual voice.

The digitized dictation can be sent, or "farmed out," to a variety of satellite transcribers, or **transcription ports,** some of which use audiocassettes onto which the signals are converted back into voice, and others of which simply convert the signals directly into voice through an internal processor within the transcriber, without the use of a cassette tape.

Computerized voice processing machines are beneficial in that a transcription supervisor can assign various dictation to transcriptionists, dictation can be more easily identified, managed and prioritized than with a typical audiocassette transcriber, and dictation can be saved for a longer period of time and in a more compact manner than on typical audiocassettes. One drawback is that each transcriptionist must have access to a transcription port and may not be able to take cassette tapes home to transcribe on her or his own transcriber. Usually, however, large companies that employ digital dictation also furnish their transcriptionists with transcription ports; these ports usually must be returned to the company or hospital upon termination of employment.

Voice Synthesizers

A dictator's voice can not only be reduced to signals that must be decoded in order to hear, but the voice also can be synthesized. A **voice synthesizer,** also computer-based, changes oral dictation into a binary code, then reproduces the sound of the dictation as a signal that the computer can comprehend. These signals are subsequently converted directly into type within the computer's random access memory.

This process can work to greatly reduce the role of the medical transcriptionist, by directly transcribing oral dictation into a computer's memory. However, there are still numerous drawbacks to this type of system, including the continuous need for formatting, editing and proofreading, the limitations in the voice synthesizer's recognizable word bank (even though there are millions of medical terms, most systems can only recognize and synthesize 100,000 terms or less), and the inability of the voice synthesizer to convert the voice patterns of various dictators due to the previously described speech idiosyncracies such as dialects, accents and speech impediments.

Remote Dictation and Transcription Systems

Historically, medical transcription work environments adhered to the policy of **centralization,** a situation in which the dictator is in close proximity to the dictating equipment and the transcriptionist is in close proximity to the transcribing equipment, which could all be placed in a central location, such as the physicians' lounge or the medical records department of a hospital. Over the years, however, remote dictation has become increasingly popular with the advent of large medical transcription services, out-of-town transcription services, and independent transcriptionists, who work with a variety of physicians who would otherwise all dictate in various manners, using various types of audiocassettes.

The development of remote dictation and transcription have remedied these situations and are being used more and more. (Figure 2–2 shows a remote digital dictation/transcription system.) With **remote dictation,** the dictator records his or her message from a distant, or remote, location. Usually the dictator records her or

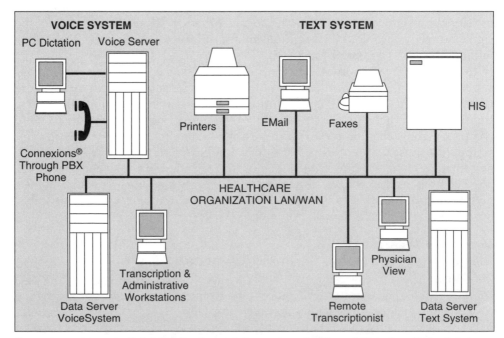

Figure 2–2   A remote digital dictation/transcription system. Courtesy of Dictaphone Voice & Data Management. Connexions® is a trademark of Dictaphone Corporation.

his dictation into a telephone; that dictation is then stored, either in a digital or an analog method, in a transcribing unit or an audiocassette tape. The dictation is then transcribed at a remote location, thus it is not necessary to return transcribed tapes.

Since the dictation is transferred to a remote location, the transcribed documents must also be transferred to the dictator's location when employing the remote method. This usually involves sending the completed **remote transcription** to the dictator via a computer and telephone, a fax or a postal delivery system.

Although the remote dictation and transcription method has many benefits, such as the ability to transcribe from remote locations, including other cities or states, and the opportunity to employ a greater variety of medical transcription services, one of its major drawbacks is that the dictator and transcriber will rarely, if ever, meet, and it is difficult to ascertain the style of the individual dictator without a lengthy trial-and-error period. Facility and format rules must be much more strictly adhered to than in an environment where the transcriptionist is in closer proximity to the dictator. Also, great care must be taken to ensure that no difficulties are encountered when transmitting work back to the dictator, because variables that are not within the transcriptionist's control, such as fallen phone lines, power surges or interruptions in power, and problems with postal or other mail delivery methods, can all serve as impediments to the timely delivering of accurate transcription.

Careful quality control mechanisms must be in place to ensure the successful outcome of optional transcription methods.

Summary of Concepts

- A transcriber, a machine that enables the transcriptionist to take oral dictation, decipher and encode it, then turn the spoken words into written material, is an essential tool for the medical transcriptionist.
- The parts of the transcriber include the control base (with play, stop, rewind, fast forward, cue and review controls), headphones and foot pedal.
- The three major types of dedicated transcribers include the standard, microcassette and mini-cassette.
- Computerized digital voice processing machines are transcribing units in which the dictator's voice is digitized into a special computer, which in turn converts the voice into digital signals and then saves them to the hard disk drive of a computer.
- Voice synthesizers change oral dictation into a binary code and then reproduce the sound of the dictation as computerized signals that are converted directly into type.
- Remote dictation and transcription involves recording dictation and performing transcription from remote (distant) locations.

Chapter 3

Telecommunications Tools in Medical Transcription

Overview: As medical transcription enters the 21st century, high-technology telecommunications tools are becoming more commonly used in the medical transcriptionist's daily work routine. Some of these telecommunications tools include state-of-the art personal computer systems; computer hardware such as Pentium processors, CD-ROMs, and expandable central processing unit (CPU) configurations; customized, easy-to-use computer word processing and operating software; and high-technology telecommunication tools such as modems, faxes, computerized bulletin boards and on-line telecommunications services. One should keep in mind, however, that equipment and technological advances will vary from workplace to workplace; for various reasons, some facilities may use only outdated, older technology, or even typewriters, while others may use only the most current technological telecommunications tools. This chapter will explore the composition, use and functionality of some of these various telecommunications tools and how they are being increasingly implemented into the medical transcriptionist's job.

Key Words

baud rate
bit
bulletin board service (BBS)
byte
CD-ROM
central processing unit (CPU)
clock speed
computer on-line service (COS)
cursor keys
cyberspace
default

disk drive
DOS (disk operating system)
downloading
DPI (dots per inch)
E-mail
fax
floppy diskette
fonts
function keys
gigabyte (gig)

graphics	monitor
hard copy	mouse
hard disk	Pentium processor
icon	peripheral device
imprint printers	personal computer (PC)
Internet	printer
keyboard	printer resolution
key-in	random access memory (RAM)
keypad	screen resolution
kilobyte (KB)	software
mainframe computer	special use keys
media	sticky-back paper
media transfer printers	telecommunications tools
megabyte (MB)	typeover
microdiskette	upgrade
microprocessor	uploading
minidiskette	Windows® software
modem	word processing

3–A Computerization and Word Processing

Computerization, the use of computers in the workplace, is now a standard part of every major industry. Medical transcription is certainly no exception. In fact, computerized word processing (keyboarding and manipulating words, or generating written communication) has become an integral part of transcribing medical reports, letters and other correspondence. Most hospitals and many physicians' offices incorporate computerization into their daily routines. Computerization is used in everything from bookkeeping to appointment scheduling to medical records production. If one is unfamiliar with it, computerization may seem frightening or intimidating at first. But with just a little familiarization with the components and uses of computer equipment, the medical transcriptionist will quickly discover that the microcomputer is one of the best pieces of equipment he or she will use. The medical transcriptionist will not only learn to like working with computers, but will also realize how limited the functions of a standard typewriter are in comparison.

Throughout this chapter various forms of equipment will be discussed. Certain pieces of equipment may be considered "outdated" or "obsolete" in today's ever-changing, high-technology world; however, keep in mind that it is important to be aware of some of these older technological methods and devices. Some facilities in which the medical transcriptionist may work or receive education may use older equipment instead of the latest technology. Reasons for not making equipment or methodology changes can range from budgetary (facilities may not be able to afford the newest equipment and technology) to preference (facilities may simply prefer what they are comfortable and familiar with rather than constantly changing equipment and methods). Oftentimes smaller or older facilities (especially schools and older hospitals and clinics) will receive used equipment from larger settings that may be purchasing new equipment or reducing their own costs (downsizing). Sometimes facilities are the recipients of donations of equipment and tools from other organizations or facilities. Thus, medical transcriptionists should not be surprised if at some point during their careers they find themselves working with what they and others may consider "obsolete" equipment.

What Is Word Processing?

Word processing, or information processing, is a clerical support system involving the use of technology, proper procedures and trained personnel in creating, compiling and maneuvering a body of written material. Historically, creating documents, medical and others, has always been rather simple: either handwriting or typewriting was used to generate text. A major problem with handwritten text is that it can be hard to decipher and is usually not uniform. This is particularly critical in medical transcription, where medical records may be legal documents, thus must be completely legible and understandable. Although many nurses' and doctors' notes are initially handwritten, they usually are transcribed in a more uniform format when placed in the permanent medical record.

The greatest difference between a typewritten document and a word-processed document is that the latter is stored and can be retrieved for making changes, corrections or additions. A typewritten document must be retyped (or "whited out" with liquid opaquing or dry erasure material, which is *never* acceptable in medical records) in order to undergo these same modifications, which consumes much more time and is a far greater inconvenience than the word processing method.

Compiling and maneuvering the information is, therefore, quite complex with handwriting and typewriting: if a change must be made, it has to be erased, corrected with opaquing fluid, or manually removed in some other way; if something must be added or moved, the entire text or a portion thereof usually has to be cut, copied, pasted and/or rekeyed.

The information processor is able to perform the tasks of creating, compiling and maneuvering text without the use of scissors, new paper, erasers or correction fluid. Another feature of the word processor is that, unlike the typewriter, it can also save an entire document or a group of documents. This data storage ability makes it possible to begin transcribing a medical record, save it, retrieve it later, and work on it again and again. Additionally, multiple copies of documents can be made at any time without the use of reproductive copiers. Therefore, word-processed medical records are more permanent, flexible and easily manipulated than typewritten or handwritten medical records.

What Are Microcomputers?

Microcomputers, often called **personal computers,** or **PCs,** are quite a bit smaller than their **mainframe computer** predecessors, which took up large portions of offices and were cumbersome and extremely complicated to use. Microcomputers use disks or diskettes to store information. Large microcomputer systems with large memory banks also use audiocassette tapes as backup systems.

You may often hear the terms *PC* and *word processor* interchanged, however, word processing involves only one of the many functions of personal computers. Word processing software programs such as WordPerfect®, Microsoft Word®,

Microsoft Write® and WordStar® contain instructions, procedures and formats for easy keyboarding. Some programs that are used to perform other computer functions have word processing programs (such as Microsoft Works®) included as well. Unlike a typewriter, a word processing program allows one to print bold type, italics and double underlining, to print different type styles **(fonts)** to print **graphics** such as pictures, boxes, complex designs, and charts, and to perform a variety of other functions that would be difficult or impossible on a regular typewriter. These functions can be important to a medical transcriptionist, because a dictator often will ask for a word or phrase to be underscored or italicized. For example, when listed in a medical record, allergies oftentimes are keyed in bold type. A simple typewriter probably would not be able to perform such a basic but necessary function.

Most PCs, in addition to information processing, also allow the user to perform other tasks, such as creating and maintaining databases and spreadsheets. Databases are documents that are comprised of large pieces of raw data, such as patient names, birth dates, medical record numbers, diagnoses, and so on. Databases often are used in medical settings such as billing and medical information/data processing departments. Spreadsheets are electronic worksheets, often complex tables containing numbers and formulas. They frequently are used in medical billing departments and in the front offices of medical offices and clinics to prepare patient financial information and maintain bookkeeping records.

3–B PC Components: Hardware

A PC, at the very least, consists of a monitor, a keyboard, and a CPU. (Figure 3–1 shows the major components of a personal computer.) Peripheral devices such as printers are discussed later. The medical transcriptionist should become familiar

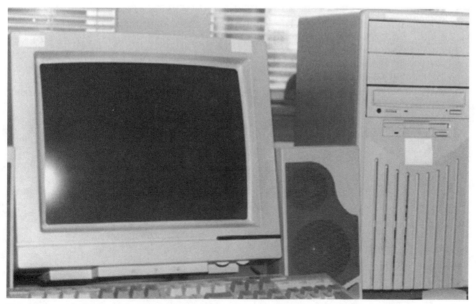

Figure 3–1 The Personal Computer (PC)

with the various types of PC hardware used in medical facilities, as well as the terminology.

The Monitor

The **monitor** is the component of the computer also known as the screen. On the monitor, work is viewed as it is keyed in, similar to seeing the words on paper when working on a typewriter. (See the later section "A Note on Color.") Monitors usually display what is keyed in one of four types of image quality, or **screen resolution:** MGA (monochrome graphics adaptation, or one color, such as green, blue or amber, and black and the single-color shading techniques), CGA (color graphics adaptation, with 16 of the major colors such as green, magenta, blue and black, and a variety of shading techniques), VGA (video graphics adaptation, with 256 colors and an unlimited amount of black and color shading techniques), or SVGA (super video graphics adaptation, containing everything the VGA monitor does but at a higher resolution, or the amount of dots, or pixels, used in generating an image on the monitor). The higher the resolution of a monitor, the lower the dot pitch, which usually is measured in millimeters (e.g., an image displayed on a 0.25 DP monitor has a higher resolution and greater definition than an image displayed on a 0.55 DP monitor). A monitor with higher resolution is easier on the eyes than a lower-resolution monitor, which is important when viewing the medical reports one transcribes.

The Keyboard

You probably are already familiar with the **keyboard.** This is the part of the computer on which you **key-in,** or type, characters. There are two major types of keyboards: the older IBM 10-function keyboard and the more common enhanced IBM 12-function keyboard. Figure 3–2 shows some alternative keyboards. Most of the keys on a keyboard are quite similar to the keys of a regular typewriter. However, in addition, you will note some special keys not found on a typewriter, such as the "F1" through "F12" keys, or the **function keys,** the **cursor keys,** and the **special use keys.** The cursor keys include the ones with arrows on them, or the directional cursor keys, plus the "Home," "End," "PgUp" (or page up), and "PgDn" (or page

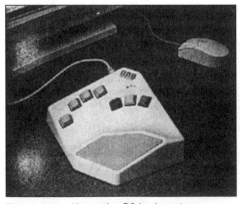
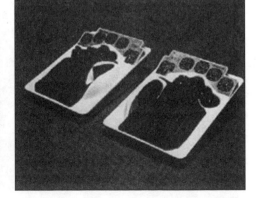

Figure 3–2   Alternative PC keyboards

down) keys. The special use keys include the "Ins" and "Del" keys (or insert and delete) keys, the "Ctrl" and "Alt" keys (or control and alternate) keys, and the "Esc" (or escape) key.

The keyboard also contains a group of numbers, called a **keypad,** which allows one to perform 10-key (adding machine) functions without using the numeral keys at the top of the keyboard and without using a separate calculator or adding machine. Although the keypad is not typically used when transcribing, it is important to familiarize yourself with it. The keypad numbers usually contain a duplicate set of cursor keys, including arrow keys on the numbers 2, 4, 6 and 8; the "Home," "End," "PgDn," and "PgUp" keys on 7, 1, 3 and 9, respectively; and the "Ins" and "Del" keys on the 0 and decimal (.) keys, respectively. The #5 key on the keypad does not function as a cursor key. You will notice that all of the word and arrow cursor keys are also located as separate keys between the keypad and the regular typewriter letter portion of the keyboard.

The function keys usually have specialized tasks, or functions, that vary with each word processor. Some of these functions could include underlining, boldfacing, or italicizing, spell checking, and other important mechanisms used when transcribing.

The cursor keys move your cursor (usually a flashing bar that tells you where your next character will be keyed) around a page or document. With the cursor arrow keys, you can move your cursor to the left, to the right, and up and down. You can also move the cursor a great distance at a time, such as an entire page or to the very beginning or very end of a document, no matter how many pages it contains.

The special use keys allow you to manipulate text and controls in a manner unavailable on typewriters. The control and alternate keys usually allow the function or other keys to have a third and fourth level of functioning (the first level is the key by itself, the second level is the key with "Shift" depressed). The insert key allows you to switch off and on, or toggle, the modes of inserting text. These modes are called insert and **typeover.** In the typeover mode, at the point marked by a flashing bar or other character representing a placeholder (the cursor), text is typed over and replaced concurrently with new text. In the insert mode, at the cursor, new text is inserted into existing text. The **default** (standard settings that exist before changing) setting for the insert key is usually in the insert mode, to prevent accidental erasure of text. You will probably want to keep your PC in the insert mode when transcribing, so as not to replace important information already keyed in. The delete key is similar to the regular backspace key on the typewriter; however, it deletes characters to the right or in front of the cursor instead of deleting characters behind or to the left of the cursor, as does a typical typewriter backspace key.

Last is the "Enter" key, which performs the same task as the "Return" key on a regular typewriter.

The CPU

Another part of the microcomputer hardware is the **central processing unit (CPU),** which is the "brain" of the microcomputer. The CPU configuration, or design, can either be in a flat, base unit format, or in a stacked, tower or mini-tower format. The disk drives, CD-ROM ports and various other peripherals are located within or attached to the CPU.

There are many types of CPUs on the market today, but each contains a minimum number of operating mechanisms, or specifications. Minimally, these specifications include the type of microprocessor (also called processor), the clock speed, the amount of memory (random access memory, or RAM), disk drives, operating systems, and various other peripherally related mechanisms such as the mouse, joysticks, graphics drivers, serial or parallel ports, and printers (discussed later).

The Microprocessor, Clock Speed and BUS One of the most important components of the CPU is the **microprocessor,** or brain, of the CPU. The microprocessor usually is one of the following types: a **Pentium processor,** which is really a high-performance 586 or 686 speed microprocessor, a 486 DX or SX microprocessor, a 386 DX or SX microprocessor, or a 286 microprocessor (these were among the first types of microprocessors contained in CPUs and are now rarely found).

Another main feature of the CPU is the **clock speed.** The speed of the internal clock (not the regular clock that keeps time, but the device that measures the speed at which the microprocessor functions) is measured in megahertz, or mHZ, such as 25, 33, 50 or 66 mHZ, or at Pentium speeds of 75, 90 or 133 mHZ, and greater.

Another CPU feature, the BUS, is the main data transmission line that sends all data and instructions from one portion of the CPU or operating system to another.

Random Access Memory The **random access memory** (or **RAM**), also known as the "memory" of the computer, is the portion of the CPU that is reserved for holding temporary instructions used in programs, holding temporary data being manipulated, and storing temporary data. The more RAM a CPU contains, the more complex programs the CPU can run without compromising other functions such as printing, saving, or working concurrently in other programs. The RAM allows you to perform certain functions without having to access the main operating system and also "remembers" certain things without you having entered, retrieved, or saved them previously.

Measured in **megabytes (MB),** RAM usually comes in multiples of four (although older 286 processors and some 386 processors only came with 1 or 2 MB of RAM). Typical increments of RAM include 4 MB, 8 MB, 16 MB and 32 MB. Most RAM is expandable up to hundreds of megabytes, although usually a small amount of RAM is included with the standard CPU. The switches that turn the computer off and on are also generally located on the CPU.

Disk Drives As the RAM is the major memory component of the CPU, the **disk drives** are the major storage components. The drives themselves are devices that actually spin disks, both the hard disk that is internal to the computer (and in most cases nonremovable) and one or more removable floppy (so named because the first floppy diskettes were actually "floppy" and were bendable and therefore highly damageable) diskettes. **Floppy diskettes** are removable square plastic containers housing circular, or disk-shaped, devices on which computerized data can be stored. You should store medical records you have transcribed onto floppy diskettes on a regular basis. Floppy diskettes come in two sizes—the standard **microdiskette** (3½-inch) and the older and less commonly used **minidiskette** (5¼-inch). Most newer PCs that come factory-prepared only have drives that accept the microdiskette, although many frequently have empty slots that you can

upgrade (update or renovate) to house the larger minidiskette so older programs and documents created and saved on these diskettes can be used.

By spinning the disks, the drives allow both the transferring of data to (data writing) and extracting data from (data reading) a disk or diskette. The drives also function to provide correct timing of movement of the surface, or lateral head, of the disk or diskette, and allow the disk or diskette to move to the correct position for reading or writing (called sector). The external drives contain an opening, or slot, into which a diskette is put, and a button, lever, or door, which when in the closed and locked position informs the CPU that the diskette is ready to be read or written to.

Disk drives usually are indicated in writing with a designation of a capital letter, followed by a colon, such as C:. Usually, the drive labels A: and B: are reserved for floppy diskette drives; drive labels C:, D:, E: and above, are used to indicate hard disk drives, CD (compact disk) drives, or other internal and typically nonremovable CPU drives.

The **hard disk** is a nonremovable internal disk located within a metal cabinet in the inner portions of the CPU. Because the hard disk is used to store the majority of programs, instructions, operating systems, and documents that need to be permanently placed within the confines of the CPU, capacity for storage is very important when selecting a hard drive to meet the needs of the PC operator. Usually, very few programs use a large amount of hard drive space (RAM is much more important in this regard); however, each program uses some space, and when documents are added, the operating system is in place and consideration is taken regarding free disk space, thus a large capacity hard drive is a necessary requirement.

As previously stated, computers use the binary system (a mathematical system using only the digits 0 and 1 as opposed to the digits 0, 1, 2, 3, 4, 5, 6, 7, 8 and 9, used in the decimal system). A single number, either a "0" or "1", is called a **bit** in computer language. Eight bits together are known as a **byte,** which is the most common informational unit used in computer terminology. Disk capacity is measured in bytes, and multiples of bytes, such as **kilobytes,** megabytes and **gigabytes.** (See Table 3–1, Byte Measurement Conversion.)

While a hard disk usually minimally contains 100 or 200 MB, and optimally 1 gig or more of storage space, a floppy diskette usually has the maximum capacity of

---

Table 3–1   Byte Measurement Conversion

---

1 byte = approximately 0.67 information pieces (characters or character spaces)

1 character = approximately 1.5 bytes

1 byte = 8 bits (eight 0s or 1s, such as 00110010, in binary language)

1 kilobyte (1 KB or Kb) = approximately 1,000 bytes

1 megabyte (1 MB or Mb) = 1 million bytes

1 gigabyte (1 gig) = 1,000 megabytes or 1 billion bytes

1.44 MB of storage space, which is a high-density value; a low-density diskette has a maximum capacity of 360 KB of storage space. Even with a large hard disk, several floppy diskettes are always needed for saving, backup and utility purposes. A good rule of thumb is that for every MB of hard drive storage capacity you need (for example, 80 MB), double that value (160 MB) and add 100 MB (260 MB) to ensure that the hard drive will be large enough so it will not be outgrown too quickly. Also, you should have one-sixth of the amount of floppy diskettes (in the previous example, with a 260 MB hard drive you would need at least 43 MB in diskettes, or about 30 floppy diskettes) on hand for storage, backup and utility purposes.

Although the majority of hard disks are still nonremovable, a newer, removable hard disk is being used in conjunction with computerized digital medical dictation and transcription systems. Also, high-capacity audiocassette tape data storage units are becoming increasingly popular as substitutes for second and additional hard drives and also as backup data storage systems.

CD-ROM Drives A **CD-ROM** is an acronym for a computerized "Compact Disk, with Read Only Memory." This drive-controlled computerized device utilizes compact disks identical in form but sometimes different in function from CDs used to play music. (Most computers CD-ROM drives can play musical CDs, but musical CD players cannot read computer CDs.) A CD-ROM is placed into a drive port in the CPU case configured for graphical computer CDs. Unlike hard disks and floppy diskettes, from which programs, files and documents can be read and to which files and documents can also be saved, the contents of a CD-ROM can be read only, as the name implies, and not written to.

Some advantages a CD-ROM has over diskettes are that a CD-ROM is more durable than an ordinary floppy diskette, it is more mobile than a permanent hard disk contained within a CPU, and it can hold approximately 130 MB of information, as much as a small hard drive or about 100 times as much as a floppy diskette. Some drawbacks to a CD-ROM are that currently you are not able to save information to the CD-ROM or change information contained on it, the speed of its use is somewhat slower than its disk components, and the cost is double to triple the amount of a floppy diskette with similar contents upon it. However, this cost disparity is often due to the more complex programs and graphics that can be contained on a CD-ROM due to its large information storage capacity and higher resolution than ordinary diskettes.

Now in development and soon to be in standard use are CD-Read and Write drives, which will be able to be written to as well as read and will make them as popular as floppy diskettes with a much greater storage capacity.

3-C PC Peripheral Devices

A **peripheral device,** or a component added or attached to the outside, or periphery, of a PC, is a component that is essential to the full use of the computer's word processing and other capabilities but is not usually necessary for basic operation, such as the mouse, the line printer (LPT), and the communications port(s) (COM).

The Mouse

The **mouse** is a hand-controlled device that generates electrical impulses that emulate its current location. These impulses can be seen on the monitor via a specially shaped cursor that corresponds to mouse movements. The mouse is used with a variety of Windows-based computer programs to open and use menu options for text manipulation and other features of a specific program.

The Printer

The **printer,** also called line printer, from which the abbreviation LPT derives, makes a **hard copy** (paper copy) of any data you designate to be printed. Most printers today can print with either black output (used primarily for text) or color output (used primarily for graphics). Printers can be classified in several ways, including: 1) printer resolution (in dots per inch or single stroke), 2) printer interface capability (serial or parallel port), and 3) printing medium used (imprint or media transfer). See Figure 3–3.

Printer Resolution   The **printer resolution,** or clarity or sharpness of the printed image, is important when deciding how your work will appear when printed. Printers have two major differences in resolution: those that print in some sort of dots per inch **(DPI)** resolution, and those that print in a single strike (no dots) resolution. Dot resolution printers include dot matrix printers, inkjet printers and laser-jet printers.

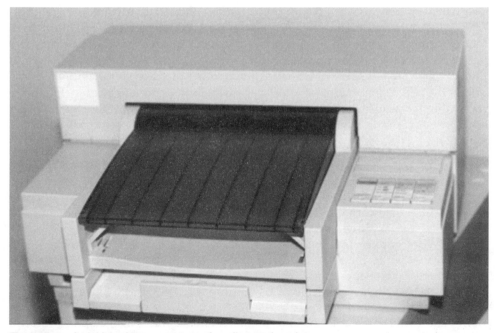

Figure 3–3   An inkjet printer—one type of media transfer printer

Dot matrix printers use an arrangement of pins that emit dots, one dot for each pin, to generate characters and graphics. Dot matrix printers commonly include 9 DPI printers, which print only in visible dot matrix form, and 24 DPI printers, where the printed output can range anywhere from a visible dot matrix form to small, almost imperceptible dots. An inkjet printer's character composition is usually a minimum of 300 DPI or greater. The dots in an inkjet printer are imperceptible. A laser-jet printer's character composition is also usually a minimum of 300 DPI or greater. The dots in a laser-jet printer are also imperceptible.

Most dot matrix and inkjet printers are low-to-medium resolution printers, as their output is usually clear but often not very sharp. Some inkjets and all laser-jets are called high-resolution printers, as the output is usually exceedingly clear and exceptionally sharp.

Another type of high-resolution printer is the daisywheel printer. It was once quite common but is now used in only a few medical transcription environments, employing the same character output as a regular typewriter—a single strike. The striking implement is one metal or plastic component versus many pins or ink dots; thus, the output of the daisywheel printer is smooth and clear, as it is with the typewriter. However, usually daisywheel printers can print far fewer types of graphics and font sizes than the more standard dot and jet printers.

Printer Interface Capability   Each printer must be connected to the CPU via a connection. There are two types of connections: software and hardware. The software connection from a computer to a printer is called a printer driver. The printer driver allows computer programs to communicate with the printer and print characters and images similar to or exactly the way they are displayed on the screen. The hardware, or physical, connection from a computer to a printer is called an interface. An interface is a device that allows the CPU to literally send information to the printer to be printed. There are two types of printer interfaces: parallel ports and serial ports. A parallel port is the most common type of port, in which eight or more signals are transmitted over an equal number of wires concurrently. A serial port is the less common type of interface, in which two or more printer signals are transmitted in sequence rather than concurrently. All types of printers can be either serial or parallel; check with your printer's manufacturer for specific details.

Printing Media   The **media** a printer uses include both the type of mechanism it uses to print characters (ribbon, ink or toner) and the kind of paper on which it prints. **Imprint printers** use ribbons or ribbonlike printing media to produce an imprint, or impression, of a character, symbol or design. Dot matrix and daisywheel printers are common types of imprint printers. Imprint printers can print on multipart (two, three or more sheets printed together) or tractor-fed paper. A tractor-feeder, or form-feeder, is a mechanism that has raised grooves and a holder to accommodate a roll or stack of paper that is continuously attached, usually with a perforation separating individual pages, with holes at the lateral edges. Medical transcription facilities that use multipart paper and/or form-fed paper employ imprint printers.

Imprint printers typically use black and multicolor pre-inked ribbons. Imprint printers primarily use lightweight bond (#24, or 24 pound, or less) paper. The heavier and thicker card stock (thin, #40, or 40 pound, or greater) usually does not work well with imprint printers. The special **"sticky-back" paper** used in a majority of physician's offices for office notes (usually a thick bond with an adhesive coating on the obverse side) is also usually not compatible with imprint printers. Most imprint printers can print through several pages of multipart paper, although the quality of the printing is usually best on the first page and diminishes on the second and subsequent pages. Printing single sheets or envelopes on imprint printers can be facilitated with a special feeding device, although some types of imprint printers cannot accommodate nonstandard sizes of paper such as envelopes.

Media transfer papers use a transfer process to move print media such as ink or toner to the paper. Two of the most commonly used media transfer printers in medical transcription environments are inkjet printers and laser-jet printers. Inkjet printers use a liquid ink that is dispensed through minute holes from a cartridge, tube or other container. The ink is forced through the holes in the container, forming small, highly accurate jets as the ink is projected onto the paper. The ink is usually permanent, is somewhat water-resistant, and is available in black and the major computer colors (see the following section "A Note on Color"). Inkjets print best on bond paper. Some models do accommodate card stock and sticky-back paper, but few, if any, can print on continuous or multipart paper. Unless a special tray, lever or adaptor is provided for printing envelopes, this process can be frustrating, if not impossible.

Laser-jet printers use a dry black powder called toner, which is dispensed from a large cartridge, similar to that of a photocopier. The laser-jet, also like the photocopier, "burns" the toner onto the paper with the aid of a laser mechanism, permanently affixing the toner to the paper. The toner in laser printers, like inkjet printers, forms jets as the toner is projected onto the paper. Again, some models do accommodate card stock and sticky-back paper, but few, if any, can print on continuous or multipart paper, and as with inkjets, unless a special tray, lever or adaptor is provided for printing envelopes, this process can be difficult or impossible.

Daisywheel printers are the printers most similar to typewriters. The major differences between a daisywheel printer and a typewriter that uses a daisywheel is that 1) the printer is connected to a computer and the typewriter is not (although some advanced typewriters do have a serial port for connection to a computer), and 2) the daisywheel printer usually prints at a higher rate of speed than does the typewriter. Daisywheel printers use an inked ribbon printing media, and they use a single strike for each character. Usually all types of paper can be accommodated by the daisywheel, whether it is bond, card stock, sticky-back, multiform or continuous. Envelopes usually can be printed on a daisywheel printer, although unless there is a special feeder specifically for them, they may have to be hand-fed individually. Some daisywheel printers can perform multicolor printing, but most do not support graphics, thus multicolor printing is less useful in these types of printers than others.

3-D A Note on Color

Two types of colors are used in computers, screen colors and printer colors. Screens were once monochrome, displaying images only in the various shades of black and one other color (such as green or amber). Now images can be displayed in 256 different shades. This is an important concept for the medical transcriptionist, as it is important for someone who spends a great deal of time in front of a computer screen to choose a screen color that will minimize eye fatigue.

Formerly, computer printers printed only one color: black. Complex graphics, designs and pictures were not an option to be either displayed or printed on a computer. Now, however, graphics are the rule rather than the exception in PC use. Graphics such as pie charts, graphs and charts are sometimes incorporated into medical reports and scientific papers. Additionally, forms, flyers, letterhead and photographs, all necessitating the use of color, are becoming more commonly used in various medical transcription environments. In order to use these richly multicolored graphics, color must be able to be recognized on the screen and printed on the page.

Color works in two separate ways on the monitor and with the printer. On the computer screen, color is displayed through a variety of three major color values: red, green and blue (abbreviated RGB). Each of these minute monitor color components is called a phosphor. Three phosphors arranged together comprise a pixel, derived from "picture element"—the smallest unit of light that can be displayed on a computer monitor. From the three phosphors, eight "basic" pixel colors can be formed, by combining none, one, two or three phosphors into a pixel.

Varying the intensity and position of these eight pixel colors—black, white, red, green, blue, cyan, magenta and yellow—produces the various shades and combinations of these colors that constitute the 256 colors that can be displayed on a color monitor. Because the pixel intensities are combined or added to form different colors, screen color is called an additive process.

Ink color, when used in printing, uses a subtractive process. The intensity of the three major ink colors—cyan, yellow and magenta (abbreviated CYM)—is subtracted to form the same 256 colors that can be displayed on the computer screen. In this case, black printer ink is an equal mixture of all three ink colors—cyan, yellow and magenta. (This is composite black ink; some printers also use a separate, strictly black ink.) As colors are subtracted from composite black, the various 256 colors are formed. The white ink of a printer really is the absence of all ink colors, or the "white page" (or whatever color your paper medium is).

Like screen colors, from the three basic ink colors, eight "basic" ink colors can be formed, by subtracting various amounts of ink from composite black.

Unlike the screen display, a printer can actually only print these eight colors. The printer uses techniques called pattern and scatter to produce the remaining shades of color that can be displayed on the screen. This process is called half-toning. In pattern half-toning, the printer driver produces a larger pixel than the one visible on the screen called a dither cell. More shades of color than are possible in one pixel can be formed in a dither cell, and the dither cell can be reduced or enlarged to create colors identical to screen colors. Scatter half-toning works similarly to pattern half-toning, except that instead of using dither cells, fragments of the color found in screen pixels are randomly placed on an indicated section of paper, which lessens the geometric color dots often seen with pattern half-toning.

When displaying or printing an image exclusively in black and white, color values are represented in shades of gray. This manner of expression of color is called gray-scale.

3–E PC Software

Personal computers use program packages, or applications, known as **software.** These applications include programs that perform functions such as systems operation, word processing, database processing, spreadsheet processing, graphic arts generation, desktop publishing, game-playing, and so on. Software is comprised of floppy diskettes or CD-ROMs (which contain the programming), instructional and reference manuals, and materials such as templates (paper or plastic overlays for the keys that explain the role of the keys, especially the function keys, and other uses of the keyboard for a particular software program). Some software runs on an individual computer (called dedicated software) and other programs run on a central or mainframe computer connected to other satellite computers that can use the portions of the software, usually without being able to make major configuration changes to the central computer (called network software).

Systems Operations Software and Windows

There generally have been two types of microcomputers used over the past decade, when computers became so popular for home use: the Apple® computer varieties (now more commonly known as MacIntosh®) and the IBM-compatibles (with common brand names such as IBM®, Packard Bell®, Hewlett-Packard®, Compaq®, Digital®, Acer®, AST®, etc.). The Apple® computer was developed as a visual menu-driven platform, or method of system operation. The original Apple® was easy to operate for most users in educational settings, but difficult to add many hardware and software accessories to.

The original IBM® computer, and the offspring of IBM technology, which came to be known as IBM-compatibles, ran on a DOS-based platform. Anyone who operated, or used, the PC system, had to be familiar with **DOS,** or disk operating system software, to manage documents (also called files), applications (computer programs), or the computer system itself. The DOS incorporates computer terminology, of which the user must have command to efficiently operate. Basic DOS commands such as "copy," "erase" and "move" are easy in function as well as in use, but more difficult commands such as "format," "copydisk" and "rename" are sometimes difficult concepts to grasp. Because DOS presented a challenge to users who only had to minimally operate the main computer system, computer programmers created an operating system based on DOS, but one that did not rely on DOS commands for operation, called **Windows**®, a system more similar to the Apple® computer system.

With the Windows® program, the operator uses and manipulates "windows" that contain system operating messages instead of typing in commands at the prompt. Windows® is a menu-driven program that helps the user manage both applications and files. These windows offer a selection of options which the user can choose to carry out a task, such as getting into a word processing program, operating a database program, creating a spreadsheet, using a game program, and so on. To use programs or manage or work with files and documents, you access a window or something within a window. For example, instead of typing "WP" to run your word processing program, as you might do in the DOS environment, you would simply select a small graphical representation **(icon)** contained within the window that represents your program.

A "window" in the Windows® program is actually a box or rectangle that contains several other items that allow you to create and manage applications and work space. These items can be selected by using a pointing and clicking device (typically a mouse, discussed earlier) or the ALT key, pressed simultaneously with another key. A "window" includes the following parts:

Control Menu Box   The control menu box is a small box in the upper left-hand corner of the main box that contains a minus sign (–). The control menu box allows you to resize, move, open, close, and otherwise manipulate the window.

Title Bar and Window Title   The title bar is a colored or shaded rectangular area at the top of the window. The title bar contains the window title, or the name of the application or document associated with the window. When more than one window is open, or active, the title bar of the active window is a different color or shade than any windows that are currently inactive. Depending on the nature of the window, the window title can be the name of a document, a group of documents, a directory or a file.

Menu Bar   The menu bar is a rectangular box situated under the title bar, usually uncolored, which contains a list of the available menu items. A menu item is a word that represents a choice, command, or action that can be carried out. The most commonly listed menu items are "File," "Edit," "Window" and "Help." The menu bar may also contain other menu items specific to the program or window you are using. Usually the first letter of the menu item is underscored. The menu item can either be chosen by pointing and clicking on that item or by depressing the ALT key along with the underscored character. The menu item will contain a submenu of other items configured and accessed in the same way as the main menu items.

Minimize and Maximize Buttons   These buttons are located at the upper right-hand corner of the window. The minimize button contains a downward pointing black triangle. The maximize button contains an upward pointing black triangle. The minimize button allows you to reduce the window in which you are working to an icon. Clicking on the maximize button enlarges the window in which you are working to fill the entire screen.

Scroll Bars   The scroll bars are two bars, usually gray in color, located at the right side and bottom of a window containing a movable, small square button somewhere within the bar and two directional arrow buttons. The scroll bar allows you to move parts of a document into view when the entire document will not fit on the screen at one time. The side-to-side scroll bar allows you to move from left to right; the up-and-down scroll bar allows you to move up and down within the document.

Restore Button   The restore button is a button containing two triangles, one pointing up and another pointing down, that comes into view after the maximize button is activated, when the document has become enlarged. Clicking on this button with the mouse will restore the window to its previous preenlargement size.

Window Borders   The window borders are the outside edges of a window. You can use the mouse to lengthen and shorten the height and width of the window. Clicking on the window corners allows you to lengthen and shorten two perpendicular sides of the window simultaneously.

Cursor and Mouse Pointer   The cursor, or insertion point, is a flashing bar that shows where you are in a document. It is a place-marker that lets you know where your text will appear when you begin keying. The mouse pointer is an arrow, a tall "I"-shaped character or another symbol that shows where your mouse is positioned in the document.

The background behind all the windows you see is called the desktop. All other applications, such as your word processing program, are represented in a window as an icon. In the Windows® program, the various icons are arranged by group. A group of similar programs (games, for example) is usually contained within one window. Each window group can contain several items, each an application, represented by an icon.

For further information about Windows®, consult a Windows® reference guide or your local computer store.

Word Processing Software

WordPerfect® and MS Word® are two types of word processing software frequently used by medical transcriptionists. In both WordPerfect® and Microsoft Word®, you can compose, enter, manipulate, edit and print text and graphics. Some WordPerfect® programs are DOS-based, and others run in the Windows® environment; all Word® programs are used in the Windows® environment.

Other computer software a medical transcriptionist is certain to find helpful in his or her practice includes the following:

Electronic medical dictionary software (such as Stedman's Electronic Medical Dictionary)

Electronic medical spell-checking lists software (such as Stedman's Plus)

Drug and medical terminology catalogue software (such as Stedman's Word-Watcher)

Computer-aided translation (CAT) [medical shorthand] and abbreviations software (such as IntelliCAT and PRD Plus)

Bookkeeping and accounting software (such as Quicken)

Calendar and organizational software (such as Lotus Organizer)

For further examples of types and uses of software, consult the instructional materials provided with the PC you are using or your nearest computer software retail store or library.

3–F Other Telecommunications Tools

Telecommunications tools are devices that use telephone cables or wires, and even the air waves, to help us communicate. These tools include high-tech computers, telephones, and more recent so-called "super-telecommunications tools" such as cellular phones, modems, faxes and computer bulletin boards. Telecommunications tools have always been used in medical transcription, and with the advent of super-telecommunications, the tools utilizing these processes are gaining even more widespread use in current times. Some tools that are becoming more commonly used in medical transcription will be briefly discussed next.

Modems   A **modem** is a shortened word form/acronym for modulator-demodulator. A modem is necessary for a computer to communicate with other computer systems. Remote dictation and transcription would be impossible without modems. A modem can be internal (installed inside the CPU) or external (located outside the CPU and attached to it through an external port). Modems are peripheral computer devices that sequentially transmit data from one computer to another over telephone lines or air waves. (Using a modem typically requires two phone lines: one for regular telephone conversations, and a second noninterruptable phone line—without features such as call waiting—for modem and/or facsimile connections.) Transmission of data includes **uploading** (sending data to a PC) and **downloading** (receiving data from another PC). Data is transmitted at a rate called a **baud rate;** the faster the baud rate, the faster the data is transmitted. A baud is equivalent to one telecommunications beat, or pulse, per second.

Typical modem baud rates are 1200, 2400, 9600, 14400, 28800, 36600, 48800, 54400, and higher pulses per second. A 28,800 byte document (230,400 bits) would theoretically take approximately eight seconds to be transmitted from one computer to another with a 28800 baud modem, while a 2400 baud modem transmitting the same information would take approximately three minutes. However, you must realize that the speed at which your PC communicates with the other PC also is dependent upon its speed. If it is transmitting and/or receiving data at a lower rate than your PC, expect delays in sending and receiving information.

Other modem specifications include data bits (measured in 5, 6, 7, or 8), stop bits (measured in 1, 1.5, or 2), parity (indicated as none, odd, or even), flow control, and connector (which specifies which communications port, or COM, the modem is transmitting through—usually COM1 or COM2). Modems can be of great use in remote dictation and transcription of medical records.

Faxes   A **fax,** a shortened word for facsimile, is a device that allows printed information to be transmitted from one location to another over telephone lines or air waves. A fax can be a dedicated fax, which is a machine that does not help compose but sends and receives hard copy pages of a document, or a fax/modem, which is a device and the related software contained within the CPU of a computer that sends and receives computerized data in the form of pages of a document. The dedicated fax only uses phone lines or air waves with the fax hardware; the fax/modem only uses the modem and phone lines/air waves when sending data and uses the modem and phone (or air waves) in conjunction with the printer when receiving data. Like modems, faxes often play a large role in remote dictation and transcription. (Figure 3–4 shows a dedicated fax machine.)

Computer Bulletin Boards   Just as medical transcriptionists work in a specialized environment—a hospital, a doctor's office, a service, or a home environment—

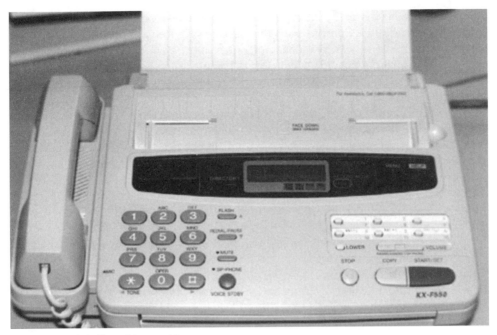

Figure 3–4   A dedicated fax machine

computers communicate in a specialized environment. This environment, in which modems exchange pulse rates, faxes receive carefully crafted pages and graphics, and telephone lines remain ever-busy, is called **cyberspace**—the intangible and infinite universe of telecommunications. One feature of this unseen universe is a computer **bulletin board service,** or **BBS,** which is a computerized posting of messages, information and data available for uploading or downloading. Bulletin board services usually are set up and maintained by individuals who have an interest in a particular subject contained on the bulletin boards. Most BBSs do not charge a fee for use, other than those associated with telephone communications, such as long distance calls.

Medical transcriptionists use BBSs to post information pertinent to their profession, to upload and download files and documents, and sometimes as a "cyberport" for sending and receiving remote dictation and transcription. One could find just about anything on a BBS, from cyberspace discussions of difficult medical terminology to advertisements for transcription services available or needed. Mail can even be received via a BBS. This cyberspace mail is called **E-mail,** or electronic mail. It can be correspondence, graphics or other literature sent electronically by a computer from one cyberspace location to another and can be printed to look just like the contents of a postal envelope. An E-mail package—an entire document— also can be received from someone halfway around the world in just seconds, delivered electronically.

Computer On-Line Services   Being on-line means being connected to and ready to work with a computer. **Computer on-line services (COSs)** are commercial services that provide customers with a constant link to worldwide telecommunications. Like the BBSs, COSs provide focal points for messages, information and other data available to the user for uploading and downloading. On-line services, however, unlike BBSs, are owned by companies such as America Online, CompuServe, Delphi, GEnie, and Prodigy, for-profit companies that charge a monthly or per-item usage fee. In exchange for this fee, COSs provide all of the services that a bulletin board service offers, in addition to a variety of other products and features, including: on-line discussion (cyber "chat") areas; access to the **Internet** (initially established as a communications atmosphere for government and educational entities, and now a worldwide network of information, discussions, and vocational and avocational interests); cyberspace shopping; E-mail; and millions of other computer-based services.

Like BBSs, medical transcriptionists will find that COSs can serve as a valuable source for medical transcription information, for discussions, both professional and personal, and as a forum for exploring the intricacies of the profession such as the existence and location of educational and vocational opportunities, the pros and cons of new technology, and the differences in pay rates for medical transcriptionists nationally and worldwide.

Summary of Concepts

- Computerized word processing is now a standard part of the medical transcription industry.
- A word processor can be used to create, compile and maneuver text without the use of scissors, newspaper, erasers or correction fluid; it also has the ability to save and retrieve documents.
- Most computers used in offices and hospitals today are called microcomputers, or PCs.
- A PC's hardware consists of, minimally, a monitor, keyboard and CPU.
- The monitor, or screen, displays what one is keying or what has been previously keyed on the PC.
- The keyboard, from which one types, or keys-in, characters, consists of a variety of keys, including function keys, cursor keys, special use keys and a numerical keypad.
- The CPU, or central processing unit, is the "brain" of the computer.
- The microprocessor is the brain of the CPU.
- Random access memory, or RAM, the "memory" of the computer, holds temporary program instructions and temporary data as well as stores temporary data.
- Disk drives are the major storage components of the CPU.
- Floppy diskettes are removable square plastic containers housing circular, or disk-shaped, devices on which computerized data can be stored.
- A hard disk is a nonremovable internal disk located within a metal cabinet in the inner portions of the CPU, which has a high capacity for data storage.

- Bytes are the basic unit of computer data; bytes are further broken down into kilo-bytes (1,000 bytes), megabytes (1 million bytes) and gigabytes (1,000 megabytes).
- A CD-ROM is a special computerized compact disk that is removable, is more durable than floppy diskettes, and has a large capacity for storage.
- Peripheral devices include those such as a mouse, a printer and communications ports.
- There are two major types of printers—imprint printers, such as dot matrix and daisywheel printers, and transfer printers, such as inkjet and laser-jet printers.
- Printer media, including the type of printing mechanism used (ribbon, ink or toner) and the type of paper that can be used in the printer, are important factors when considering which printer to use in medical transcription.
- Computer screen colors are composed of three color phosphors (red, green and blue), which can be varied in intensity and added to form pixels, the major picture element of the screen; printer screen colors are composed of three main ink colors (cyan, yellow and magenta), which can be combined with various methods and subtracted to form the remaining 256 computer color shades.
- PCs use program packages known as software, which allow the user to perform functions such as systems operation, word processing and graphic arts generation.
- Telecommunications tools such as modems, faxes, computer bulletin boards and computer on-line services help medical transcriptionists communicate, access information, and receive electronic mail (E-mail).

Chapter 4

Use of Reference Materials

Overview: Some additional important tools medical transcriptionists use on a daily basis are reference materials such as dictionaries, texts, indices, word lists, and other books and written materials to aid in choosing a correct word and correctly spelling that word. This chapter contains some helpful and frequently used reference materials, which should be added to the medical transcriptionist's personal library over time.

Key Words

drug index/catalogue

grammar reference book

medical dictionary

medical specialty word book

medical word book

4–A Types of Reference Materials

A medical transcriptionist uses many types of reference materials to practice in his or her field. Some of the major types of medical transcription references, as well as their use and examples of each, are detailed next.

Reference Book Types

Medical Dictionary   Look up words in this book in overall alphabetical order. Look up double words (such as Hemophilus influenzae) by either the first or last word. This gives a complete definition of all words. Examples include *Dorland's Medical Dictionary, Mosby's Medical Dictionary, Stedman's Medical Dictionary*, and *Taber's Cyclopedic Medical Dictionary.*

Drug Index/Catalogue   Look up drug and medicinal names in one of several ways: alphabetically, by product (trade) name, generic (common) name, manufacturer's index (maker's name), or product category (systemic use of drug, e.g., antipruritic), or any combination of the preceding. Examples include *Physicians' Desk Reference (PDR), Billups' American Drug Index*, and *The Pill Book.*

Transcription Style Guide　Look up questions you might have about medical transcription style, formats, and mechanics of abbreviations, numerals, capitalization, punctuation types, and so on. Look up questions by various categories. This guide usually includes sections on often misspelled/misused words. Examples include *The Medical Transcriptionist Handbook, The Do's and Don't's of Medical Transcription,* and *The AAMT Style Guide in Medical Transcription.*

Medical Word Book　There are two major types of medical word books. In one, the systemic word listing guide, a word is looked up in the section dealing with its associated system (i.e., for retinitis you would look in the ophthalmology section). In the other type, the alphabetical word listing guide, a word is looked up in its overall alphabetical order. A medical word book also may contain plate diagrams of certain systems and a small number of the most frequently used drug names, surgical words, general medical words and abbreviations. Examples include *The Medical and Health Sciences Word Book, The Medical Word Book* and *Webster's Medical Speller.*

Medical Specialty Word Book　A must for the transcriptionist who transcribes specialty (systemic) medical reports, such as operative or pathology reports. Look up a word either in overall alphabetical order or by general type of instrument, operation or item (i.e., for McBurney incision, you could look under McBurney or "incision") in the surgical word book or by the specific disease name in the pathology word book. Examples include *A Word Book in Pathology and Laboratory Medicine, A Word Book in Radiology Medicine,* and *The Surgical Word Book.*

Grammar Reference Book　Look up punctuation, grammar usage, spelling rules and mechanics such as capitalization, numbers and italics first in the table of contents or index, or in the end sheets in the back of the book, and then in the page(s) to which it directs you. Examples include *The Little, Brown Handbook, The Merriam-Webster Concise Handbook for Writers, Write Right!* and *Gregg Reference.*

4-B How to Build Your Own Reference Library

A medical transcriptionist must have countless reference books and materials at his or her disposal, no matter which environment he or she works within. Some facilities will provide references for their transcriptionists; others ask transcriptionists to supply their own references. In both cases, it is helpful for transcriptionists to have a home library that can be used for study, reference and continuing education.

Some general guidelines for building and maintaining your personal medical reference library follow.

1. *Start slowly.* Do not attempt to purchase every type of reference listed in this chapter when you are beginning your career. Start with the books used in your medical transcription studies, such as medical terminology, anatomy and physiology, and pharmacology texts. You probably will already have purchased a basic medical dictionary and an English dictionary by the time you begin your first job as a transcriptionist. After a couple of months you may add a general medical word book. Two months later or so you may want to add a

specialty word book or two to your collection. You may find a grammar or style reference helpful later on as well. More books can be added as the need arises.

2. *Do not limit your reference library to books.* Use handouts, lists, and other notes as part of your library. You may want to purchase a three-ring or other bound type of folder in which you can add handouts, terminology lists, class notes, critiques given by your instructors or supervisors, and other documents that are not previously bound. You may want to alphabetize, date and label the binders and file them in a method that works for you.

3. *Used can be just as good as new.* Medical reference books are often big, bulky and expensive. Many reference books, such as dictionaries, drug catalogues, and word books, are published every one or two years. It would not only be cost-prohibitive, but exhausting to have to constantly replace your outdated references with new ones. A general rule would be to replace outdated books every three years or so. However, you may find when starting your library that a book a hospital, clinic or medical office has discarded may still be useful and would be a fine addition to your library until you are able to replace it with a more current edition. Some texts, such as the *American Drug Index,* have loose-leaf additions or supplements that can be purchased so you do not have to replace the entire text each year.

4. *Create a library cooperative.* You may not be able to afford to purchase an entire library full of reference materials and neither may your medical transcription colleagues. Consider pooling your resources to purchase texts for a mutually owned library. You could possess the texts you most often use, while other transcriptionists in the co-op could keep the ones they more commonly use at home. You may want to consult your local medical transcription organization chapter for additional ideas about forming a medical transcriptionist co-op.

Summary of Concepts

- Medical reference books, magazines and other texts are important tools for the medical transcriptionist.
- The medical transcriptionist should slowly build a personal reference library over time to aid in his or her practice of medical transcription.

Part Two

Medical Transcription Formats

Chapter 5

Types of Medical Reports and Formats

Overview: Just as the dictator has his or her own style and idiosyncrasies, so does the transcriptionist. One transcriptionist may transcribe a report one way, and another might choose another way entirely. However, it is necessary that medical records be uniform. To ensure that medical records always maintain the requirements of consistency, clarity and uniformity, transcriptionists must become familiar with the various forms, or formats, into which they should place the medical information they transcribe. Additionally, because physicians and others who dictate sometimes fail to break down a report into its correct sections, omit report names or section titles, or, oftentimes do not dictate necessary pieces of information, the medical transcriptionist must be able to identify titles and sections and other components of various types of reports. Medical transcriptionists must know the elements of how to precisely fit the sections of a rough or perhaps disorganized report together to construct a concise and complete final medical record.

Key Words

admitting privileges

aged reports

Assessment

auditory or aural evaluation

Consultation Report (CONS)

current reports

Description of the Surgical Procedure

Diagnostic Examination

Diagnostic Impression

Discharge Summary (DS)

Final Diagnosis

findings

format

free-form paragraph format

Gross Findings

history

History and Physical Report (H&P)

History of the Present Illness (HPI)

Hospital Course

inpatient

medical staffing department

Microscopic Findings

objective

olfactory evaluation

Operative Note or Report (OP)

outpatient

paragraph format

past medical history (PMH)

Pathological Diagnosis

Pathology Report (PATH)

physical

Physical Examination (PE)

Plan

Preoperative and Postoperative Diagnoses

Radiology Report (RAD)

Recommendations

Review of Systems (ROS)

sensory

separate line heading format

signs

stat reports

subjective

Surgical Findings

symptoms

tactile evaluation

the basic four

the basic six

turnaround time

visual evaluation

5–A Medical Record Formatting Basics

A medical transcriptionist must not only know which tools to use when transcribing, he or she must also be familiar with the proper order and organization into which the information being transcribed should be placed. Should the document be double-spaced and typed in paragraph form? Or should it be styled as a letter? These questions are matters of **format,** the arrangement of the proper shape, structure and general form of a particular document.

Because of the voluminous amount of documentation associated with patient hospital visits and stays, the majority of medical records have historically been produced in hospitals. From the moment a patient enters a hospital, whether that patient is admitted to the hospital for at least 24 hours to receive extended medical care (called an **inpatient**) or whether that patient simply receives diagnostic evaluation and/or treatment from a particular department of a hospital without staying a 24-hour period (called an **outpatient**), medical records of the hospital visit are produced to carefully document the patient's hospital encounter. Therefore, the majority of formats with which a medical transcriptionist must be familiar are used in the transcription of hospital dictation.

Each medical report has a unique format specifically tailored to make it concise, clear and uniform. Those who dictate usually follow a very general format for whatever report they are dictating, although every report varies slightly in content and form. Most medical reports are broken down into various sections, and those sections are further broken down into subsections. The sections have titles called headings, and the subsections have titles called subheadings. Dictators usually loosely follow these heading and subheading titles as guides for covering each aspect of the medical report. However, the report sections are only guidelines the dictator may or may not choose to follow when dictating a medical report.

5–B The Basic Six Hospital Reports

The two most basic hospital reports are called the **History and Physical Report (H&P)** and the **Discharge Summary (DS).** The History and Physical Report, dictated at the beginning of a patient's hospital admission, is the documentation of the initial evaluation of the patient's symptoms and physical disorders, as well as a summarization of the patient's condition and a plan for what should occur during the course of the hospitalization. The Discharge Summary, dictated at the conclusion of the hospital stay, is a summation of what transpired during the patient's hospital admission and what the outcome or potential outcome of the hospitalization was or may be.

In addition to the two most basic reports, two others are often dictated during a hospital stay: the **Operative Note** or **Report (OP)** and the **Consultation Report (CONS).** Combined with the H&P and DS, the OP and CONS constitute what is called **the basic four.** These four reports form the basis of the majority of all hospital dictation.

Sometimes reports dictated from two other hospital departments, those from the pathology department, called **Pathology Reports (PATH),** and those from the radiology department, called **Radiology Reports (RAD),** are grouped together with the basic four and are called **the basic six.** An explanation of each report of the basic six is discussed next.

The History and Physical Report

The H&P is the report generated by the admitting physician, the resident or the hospital internist upon formal admission of an inpatient. The report is broken down into two sections, the history and the physical. The **history,** or historical component of the report, is a summary of the chronological record of situations, events and other associated topics that may have contributed to the patient's admission into the hospital. The history portion of the report is sometimes called the **subjective,** because it relates to the patient's own sense or awareness of his or her condition and the circumstances surrounding it, factors which may or may not be able to be demonstrated. The main sections of the history section are entitled the **History of the Present Illness (HPI)** and the **Review of Systems (ROS),** or Systems Review.

The HPI is the patient's oral history given to the doctor concerning the onset and duration of the illness, as well as any precipitating factors the patient may associate with the condition. The HPI can also contain subsections concerning the patient's **past medical history (PMH),** which details any previous major illnesses or related conditions, any chronic illnesses, any previous hospitalizations or surgeries, any prior treatment for the current condition, and the patient's current immunization record, if associated with the illness. Other HPI subsections can include family, educational and social (such as smoking and alcohol consumption) histories, if they have contributed to the illness, any medications the patient may be taking, and any allergies the patient may have to specific medications and food products.

The review of systems is an historical review of the patient's complaints specific to each body system. The physician asks the patient about each body system, and the patient responds as to whether or not he or she has had problems associated with that system in the past. Again, being part of the history, the ROS is subjective, with the patient providing an oral account of what he or she senses are disturbances or abnormalities with each part of the body. In the ROS, the patient tells the physician about his or her **symptoms,** that is, the **sensory** perception of the illness—the characteristics of the illness perceived by the patient through sight, sound, smell, taste or touch.

The end of the ROS is the crossroad of the H&P report. Whereas the history focuses on the patient's subjective account of his or her current condition, the **physical,** or **Physical Examination (PE),** focuses on the characteristics of the illness that are **objective,** or capable of being demonstrated to the physician or others. These objective **findings,** or characteristics, of the disease, are often called **signs.** The physical examination is composed of a **visual** (what is seen) evaluation, an **auditory or aural** (what is heard) evaluation, an **olfactory** (what is sensed by the nose) evaluation, and a **tactile** (what is felt) evaluation, performed by the physician or health care provider. The physical exam is a series of comprehensive evaluations of the patient's body systems and organs, for example, the patient's height and weight, heart sounds, skin condition, nodules felt, reflex strength, body scents, and so on.

The H&P also usually contains two additional sections, one that formally assesses the patient's condition, also sometimes called the Impression, **Assessment,** or Admitting Diagnosis or Diagnoses, and another that provides a plan of action for the hospitalization, usually called the **Plan** or treatment plan.

The Discharge Summary

This report summarizes the hospitalization of the patient. The two major sections of the DS are the description of what transpired while the patient was in the hospital, or the **Hospital Course,** and the name or names of the specific disease, syndrome or condition that ultimately led to the patient's hospitalization, called the **Final Diagnosis** or Diagnoses.

The DS details the reason the patient was admitted to the hospital, the patient's history, and a review of the events that occurred during his or her hospitalization. Often included in the DS is a written review submitted about any pertinent laboratory and diagnostic test results, operations or procedures performed, medications given, and other information regarding the specifics of all medical care given to the patient as well as a brief review of the HPI and PE. Usually the physician also dictates sections regarding follow-up instructions, discharge medications, the patient's condition upon discharge, and the patient's prognosis.

The Operative Report

The OP report describes an operation or a surgical procedure—a procedure both manual (using a physician's hands) and operative (using surgical tools or instruments) for the purpose of correcting, repairing and diagnosing medical abnormalities, defects or diseases. The report usually is dictated by the surgeon or by an assistant. The main section of the OP report is the actual **Description of the Surgical Procedure,** sometimes simply called the Procedure. Usually also dictated in this report are the diagnoses before and after the operation, called the **Preoperative and Postoperative Diagnoses,** the name of the surgeon, the title and date of the procedure, the Indications for Surgery, and the **Surgical Findings,** or what was found upon the procedure being performed. Typically, this report also includes a sponge count and an estimation of the amount of blood lost during the procedure.

The OP report typically ends when the patient is taken to the recovery room, and the physician will usually state the condition of the patient upon leaving the operating room. (Special note: If a medical word ends in the suffixes -plasty, -pexy, -rrhaphy, or -tomy, the word most likely relates to a surgical procedure.)

The Consultation Report

The CONS report is requested from a specialist physician by the patient's primary or attending physician. The patient's attending physician requests a consultation because he or she would like a second opinion regarding a particular problem or diagnosis regarding the patient's problem. The main sections of this report are the dictating physician's (consultant's) **Evaluation** of the patient's condition, from the standpoint of his or her specialty, the consultant's **Impression** of the patient's condition, and the consultant's **Recommendations,** or what he or she recommends for further treatment of the patient relative to the scope of the consultant's area of expertise.

The CONS report is dictated by the consultant and it is addressed to (sent to) the attending physician. A consultation can be dictated in either a letter (correspondence) or report format. The CONS report usually also contains a date of consultation, the reason for consultation, physical and laboratory evaluation of the patient, and possibly specific diagnoses. There may also be a complimentary close at the end, such as "Thank you for this referral." The proper procedure is to include a closing such as this in the typed report.

The Pathology Report

The PATH report describes the pathological, or disease-related, findings of a sample of tissue taken. The tissue samples can be taken during surgery, a biopsy, a special procedure, or an autopsy. The autopsy is a special type of pathology report requested by the attending physician or a coroner when the cause of a patient's death may be doubtful or of special significance. The pathology report is dictated by a pathologist. The major sections of the PATH report are the **Gross Findings** and **Microscopic Findings** (cytology and histology), and the **Pathological Diagnosis** or diagnoses.

An important note here is that the pathology report is not synonymous with the laboratory data. The PATH report is a separate report describing specific disease findings and is usually limited to tissue, while laboratory data usually provide specific information regarding body fluids and their components. Also, the laboratory data section is only one part of another type of report (e.g., the H&P or the DS) and should never stand alone as the entire contents of a report.

The Radiology Reports

This report describes a diagnostic examination or procedure using radio waves or other forms of radiation. The radiology report is dictated by the radiologist. The major sections of the radiology report are the name of the **Diagnostic Examination,** the description of the diagnostic procedure, if included, the findings, or the body of the report, and the **Diagnostic Impression.** Sometimes a radiology report can consist simply of the name of the examination/procedure and the radiologist's impression.

Some major diagnostic examinations are roentgenograms (basic x-rays), CT scans (computerized tomography scans), MRI scans (magnetic resonance imaging scans), nuclear medicine procedures (such as thyroid scans and bone scans with an injection or infusion of radioactive contrast), fluoroscopic examinations, or any other visually recorded procedures performed on the patient to make a diagnosis. (Special note: If a medical word ends with one of the suffixes -scopy, -gram, or -graphy, the word probably relates to a radiologic examination.)

In addition to the previously discussed six major types of reports, other reports often are dictated about a patient, including the emergency room note, the psychiatric history, interim reports, the autopsy, and special procedures that receive the attention of an entire report, such as cardiac catheterization and esophagogastroduodenoscopy. Follow the general hospital report format outlined next as a general guideline for these reports, and include the titles of these reports in the report's header (patient and dictating information at the top of the page) or footer (patient and dictating information at the bottom of the page). Also see Chapter 7 Additional Medical Forms, Formats and Documents, for formatting other specific reports.

5–C General Formatting Rules

Some general formatting rules to follow when transcribing reports include:

1. *Consult the physician regarding the format.* Always consult the physician or medical institution for the proper format to use when performing transcription for that facility for the first time. Afterward, use the format required by the medical provider. Keep in mind that formats can vary greatly from institution to institution.
2. *For enhanced clarity, try to include section headings in reports.* If the institution you are transcribing for permits it, try to include section headings when none are dictated to clarify the report for the reader.
3. *Do not second-guess the dictator's intentions.* If an entire section or system component is omitted by the dictator, leave the section out; do not include the section simply because the format dictates it should be there. Also, do not transcribe that a system component is normal if it is not dictated as such. Some institutions use specific predesigned formats that require all system components to be included in a report, whether or not the specific component is dictated on; in those circumstances, unless otherwise dictated, use the predesigned format.
4. *Transcribe only required patient information.* Some offices and hospitals use different methods for noting patient identification, which is placed on the patient's medical record. The format examples that follow include only the patient's name and hospital number; however, some institutions may include such varied information as the patient's room number, address, phone number, Social Security number, age, religion, sex, marital status, diagnosis, and so on. Please be aware of this and include all information that the particular institution you are transcribing for requires. (Special note: If certain information used to identify the patient could potentially infringe upon the patient's rights or confidentiality, or cause harm in some way to the patient, such as a Social Security number, HIV status, and so on, do not disclose this information in a medical

record, even if dictated, unless specifically directed to do so by the facility or physician involved. Inclusion of any such information should be noted and documentation sent to the appropriate medical records administration personnel.)

5. *Always indicate who dictates and transcribes the report.* If someone other than the attending physician dictates the report, this is usually indicated somewhere in the report. In the examples that follow, this information, where applicable, is included in the footer. In the History and Physical Report and the Discharge Summary, if dictated by someone other than the attending physician, there are two signature lines—one for the attending physician and one for the dictating physician or other dictator. The Operative Report, Consultation Report, Radiology Report and Pathology Report, since these are almost always dictated by someone other than the attending physician, have only one signature line—one for the dictator. In the format examples that follow and in the majority of hospital formats used worldwide, the abbreviations "D:" and "T:" are often used, signifying the dates of dictation and transcription.

6. *Unless otherwise indicated, use the paragraph format.* With H&P reports, some institutions prefer listing system components of the Review of Systems and the Physical Examination in separate line heading format, each system beginning on a new line, while others prefer listing system components together in paragraph form. If the information is dictated free-form, that is, without section headings, it is sometimes easier to use the paragraph form. As a rule, use the separate line heading format unless directed otherwise in the H&P report and the free-form paragraph format for Discharge Summaries. What follows is an example of how the same material could be transcribed using both the **paragraph format, separate line heading format,** or **free-form paragraph format:**

Paragraph Format:
REVIEW OF SYSTEMS: Head: No history of head abnormalities, either genetic or traumatic. ENT: There are no otolaryngic complaints. Neck and throat: There is no history of neck or throat abnormalities. Extremities: The patient complains of frequent right shoulder pain that radiates down the arm. The rest of the systems review is normal.

Separate Line Heading Format:
REVIEW OF SYSTEMS:
Head: No history of head abnormalities, either genetic or traumatic.
ENT: There are no otolaryngic complaints.
Neck and throat: There is no history of neck or throat abnormalities.
Extremities: The patient complains of frequent right shoulder pain that radiates down the arm.
The rest of the review of systems is normal.

Free-form Paragraph Format:
REVIEW OF SYSTEMS: No history of head abnormalities, either genetic or traumatic. There are no otolaryngic complaints. There is no history of neck or throat abnormalities. The patient complains of frequent right shoulder pain that radiates down the arm. The rest of the systems review is normal.

5–D Specific Report Formats

The formats that follow are general guidelines for transcribing hospital medical records. Keep in mind, however, that these formats are not necessarily standard for all medical facilities; some hospitals may have different formats. Always consult the institution you are transcribing for before the actual transcription of the dictation.

Examples of the basic six medical reports are included here. All reports should be single-spaced, but double-spaced between paragraphs. Figures 5–1 and 5–2 demonstrate where to place patient information in reports. Figures 5–3 through 5–8 demonstrate the formats for the six major types of medical reports, with the patient information located in the footer. Again, keep in mind that these formats are only *general* guidelines; each hospital may employ its own specific formats for reports.

5–E Turnaround Time for Hospital Medical Reports

Turnaround time is the time it takes for the report to be dictated, transcribed and signed or verified by the physician. Hospital reports usually are divided into three classes in terms of turnaround time: stat, current and aged. **Stat reports,** such as radiology reports and pathology reports, usually have a turnaround time of 12 hours or less, as the report is probably required for other evaluation and treatment to be performed on the patient. **Current reports,** such as history and physical reports, consultations and operative notes, usually have a turnaround time of 24 hours. **Aged reports,** such as discharge summaries and emergency room notes, usually are not required in the patient's file before other measures can be taken in terms of his or her treatment, thus turnaround time on these reports is usually 72 hours. (An exception to the aged report rule is when patients are discharged or transferred to another medical facility; in this case, the reports need to be transcribed as soon as possible.)

Some hospital medical records departments have different turnaround times, some longer and some shorter. Turnaround times are crucial to ensuring that the medical record is completed on a timely basis, both for medical and legal reasons. Therefore, turnaround times can affect a physician's association and privileges with a hospital. A physician's **admitting privileges** constitute the authority a physician has to admit patients to a particular hospital. The **medical staffing department** of a hospital, that is, the department that hires staff physicians, in conjunction with the medical records department, provides and administers admitting privileges. Generally speaking, if a physician fails to meet the established turnaround deadline for dictating a report, he or she may have his or her admitting privileges suspended or revoked. Likewise, if the report is dictated on time and fails to be transcribed in a timely manner, the medical records department can be held liable for any medicolegal action resulting from the patient's medical files being incomplete.

It is important for the medical transcriptionist to be aware of turnaround times for specific reports and to meet the proper deadlines for the transcription of all dictation. Failure to meet deadlines could result in legal problems for the medical records department and/or disciplinary action being taken against the medical transcriptionist.

```
                    MERCY MEDICAL CENTER
                        300 Main Street
                      Denver, CO  80201


HISTORY: Xxxxxx. xxxxxxxxxxxxxxxxxxxxxxxxxxxxx
xxxxxxxxxxxxxxxxxxxxxxxx. Xxxxxxxxxxxxxxxxxxxxxxxxxxxxxxxx
xxxxx. Xxxxxxxxxxxxxxxxxxxxxxxxxxxxxxxxxxxxxxxxxxxxxxx.

Past History: Xxxxxxxxxxxxxxxxxxx. Xxxxxxxxxxxxxxxx.
Family history: Xxxxxxxxxxxxxxxxxxxxxx. Social history:
Xxxxxxxxxxxxxxxx. Other history: Xxxxxxxxxxxxxxxxxxxxxxxxx.

PHYSICAL EXAMINATION: Xxxxx: Xxxxxxxxxxxxxxxxxxxxxxxxxxxxx.
Xxxxxxx: Xxxxxxxxxxxxxxxxxxx. Xxxxxxxxxx: Xxxxxxxxxxxxxxxxxx
xxxxxxxxxxxxxxxxxxxxxxxxxx.

HOSPITAL COURSE: Xxxxxxxxxxxxxxxxxxxxxxxxxxx. Xxxxxxxxxxxxxxx
xxxxxxxxxxxxxxxxxxxxxxxxxxxxxxxxxxxxxxxx. Xxxxxxxxxxxxxxxxx
xxxxxxxxxxxxxxxxxxxxxxxxxxxxxxxxxxxxxxxx

FINAL DIAGNOSIS: Xxxxxxxxxxxxxxxxxxxxxxxxxxxxxxxxxx.

DISCHARGE PLAN: 1) Xxxxxxxxxxxxxxxxxxx.  2) Xxxxxxxxx.


                         _____
                           Xxxxx Xxxxx, M.D.




ATTENDING PHYSICIAN'S NAME                   PATIENT'S NAME
DICTATING PHYSICIAN'S NAME                   HOSPITAL #: XXXXXX
D: 01/01/XX
T: 01/02/XX
MD/mt

REPORT TITLE
```

Figure 5–2 General Medical Report, free-form paragraph style, with patient information in footer

```
                    MERCY MEDICAL CENTER
                        300 Main Street
                      Denver, CO  80201


REPORT TITLE

Patient Name: Xxxxx Xxxxx    Medical Record #:   XXXXX
Attending Physician: Xxxx Xxxx, M.D.  Room Number: XXX
Date of Admission: XX/XX/XX

HISTORY:
Xxxxxx.xxxxxxxxxxxxxxxxxxxxxxxxxxxxxx.  Xxxxxxxxxxxxxxxxxxxxxxxx
Xxxxxx. Xxxxxxxxxxxxxxxxxxxxxxxxxxxxxxxxxxxxxxxx.
Xxxxxx. Xxxxxxxxxxxxxxxxxxxxxxxxxxxxxxxxxxxxxxxxx.

Past History:
Xxxxxxxxxxxxxxxxxxxxxxxxxxxxxxxxxxxxxxxxxx. Xxxxxxxxxxxxxxxxx.
Xxxxxxxxxxxxxxxxxxxxxxxxxxxxxxxx.

Family history:
Xxxxxxxxxxxxxxxxxxxxxxxxxx.

Social history:
Xxxxxxxxx.   Xxxxxxxxxxxxxxxxxxxxxxxxxxxxxx

REVIEW OF SYSTEMS:
Xxxxxx: Xxxxxxxxxxxxxx. Xxxxxxxxxxxxxxxxxxxxxxxxxxxxx.
Xxxxxxxxx: Xxxxxxx. Xxxxxxxxxxxxxxxxxxxxxxx.
Xxxxxxxxx: Xxxxx.

PHYSICAL EXAMINATION:
Xxxxx: Xxxxxxxxxxxxxxxxxxxxxxxxxxxxxxxxxx.
Xxxxxxxx: Xxxxxxxxxxxxxxxxxxxxxxxxxxx.
Xxxxxxxxx: Xxxxxxxxxxxxxxxxxxx.  Xxxxxxxxxxxxxxxxxxxxxxxxxxxxxxx.

ASSESSMENT:
Xxxxxxxxxxxxxxxxxxxxxxxxxxxxxxxxxxxxxxxxxxxxxxx.

TREATMENT PLAN:
1.  Xxxxxxxxxxxxxxxxxxxxxxx.
2.  Xxxxxxxxx.

                         _____
                           Xxxxx Xxxxx, M.D.

D: 01/01/XX
T: 01/01/XX
XX/xx (Physician's initials followed by transcriptionist's
      initials)
```

Figure 5–1 General Medical Report, separate section style, with patient information in header

MERCY MEDICAL CENTER
300 Main Street
Denver, CO 80201

DATE OF ADMISSION: 10/02/XX

CHIEF COMPLAINT:
Difficulty breathing.

HISTORY OF PRESENT ILLNESS:
The patient is a 32-year-old, white, widowed woman who comes into the hospital complaining of dyspnea. She has been having these symptoms for over one month now. The patient was told in her childhood that she exhibited some asthmatic symptoms, although she has never been formally treated for same.

Past History:
She had a tonsillectomy and adenoidectomy at age 12.

Social History:
She is widowed; her husband died two years ago.

Family History:
Noncontributory.

REVIEW OF SYSTEMS:
Head, eyes, ears, nose and throat: She has a history of having upper respiratory tract infections every year. No throat pain. There is a history of a tonsilloadenoidectomy.
Chest: She has had no chest pain.
Gastrointestinal: Negative.
Extremities: Negative.
Neurologic: Negative.

PHYSICAL EXAMINATION:
General: She is a well-developed, well-nourished, white female. She is well dressed.
Vital signs: Temperature 36 degrees Celsius, respirations 24, pulse 78 and blood pressure 128/80. She is 5'6" tall. Her weight is 165 pounds.
HEENT: Normocephalic and atraumatic. Pupils equal, round and reactive to light and accommodation. Right pinna: There is some minimal swelling and edema around the ear lobe; it is nontender.

(CONTINUED)

JOHN DOE, M.D.   SMITH, HARRIET #123456-7
Dictated by: Doc Residente, D.O.
D&T: 10/02/XX | 10/04/XX | DR/mt

HISTORY AND PHYSICAL

Figure 5-3 History and Physical Report

Page 2

Nose: Mild rhinitis. The throat is clear.
Neck: Supple and nontender. There is no adenopathy or nuchal rigidity.
Chest: There are rales and rhonchi on expiration. Breath sounds are shallow.
Abdomen: Soft and nontender. Active bowel sounds. There is no hepatosplenomegaly.
Musculoskeletal: Negative.
Neurologic: Patellar reflexes are 2+. Deep tendon reflexes are 2+ bilaterally. No Babinskis. Normal motor and sensory exam.
Skin: Mucous membranes are moist. There is good axillary sweat.

IMPRESSION:
1.   Dyspnea.
2.   Asthma.
3.   Rule out pulmonary embolus.

PLAN:
Admit the patient to 2-North. Place the patient on a bronchodilator.
Dr. Melman, pulmonologist, will consult in the morning.

_____
John Doe, M.D.
Attending Physician

_____
Doc Residente, D.O.
Dictating Physician

JOHN DOE, M.D.   SMITH, HARRIET #123456-7
Dictated by: Doc Residente, D.O. | 10/03/XX | DR/mt
D&T: 10/02/XX | 10/03/XX | DR/mt

HISTORY AND PHYSICAL

Figure 5-3 continued

MERCY MEDICAL CENTER
300 Main Street
Denver, CO 80201

DATE OF ADMISSION: 10/02/XX   DATE OF DISCHARGE: 10/12/XX

HISTORY OF PRESENT ILLNESS: The patient is a 32-year-old, white, widowed woman who came into the Mercy Medical Center Emergency Room complaining of dyspnea. She had been having these symptoms for over one month. The patient was told in her childhood that she exhibited some asthmatic symptoms, although she had never been formally treated for same.

Past History: She had a tonsillectomy and adenoidectomy at age 12.

Social History: She is widowed; her husband died two years ago.

Family History: The patient has two brothers, ages 28 and 30; neither has had similar breathing problems. She has two children who are in high school. The patient's mother died of a myocardial infarction. The patient's father, who is living, has had carcinoma of the colon and a transurethral resection of the prostate, and he has a history of asthma.

PHYSICAL EXAMINATION: Normocephalic and atraumatic. Pupils were equal, round and reactive to light and accommodation. No icterus. No nystagmus. Funduscopic examination was negative. Right pinna: There was some minimal swelling and edema around the ear lobe; it was nontender. Nose: There was some mild rhinitis. The throat was clear. Neck: Supple and nontender. There was no adenopathy and no jugular venous distention. No nuchal rigidity. Chest: There were rales and rhonchi on expiration. Breath sounds were shallow. Abdomen: Soft and nontender. Active bowel sounds. There was no hepatosplenomegaly. Neurologic: Patellar reflexes were 2+. Deep tendon reflexes were 2+ bilaterally. No Babinskis. Normal motor and sensory exam.

LABORATORY DATA: A CBC showed a white count of 19,000 with a left shift, a hemoglobin of 13.4 grams percent, a hematocrit of 48 volumes percent, and platelet count of 100,000. The differential showed 3 bands, 5 lymphs, 7 monos and 3 eosinophils.

HOSPITAL COURSE: The patient was admitted to the 2-North Unit. A consultation was made by Dr. Lawrence B. Melman, of the pulmonology

(CONTINUED)

JOHN DOE, M.D.
D&T: 10/15/89 | 10/16/89 | JD/mt   SMITH, HARRIET #123456-7

DISCHARGE SUMMARY

Figure 5-4 Discharge Summary Report

Page 2

department. The differential diagnoses included the diagnosis of rule out pulmonary embolus. The following day a pulmonary angiogram was done and placement of a Swan-Ganz catheter was done. The patient tolerated the procedure well.

The patient was placed on a heparin drip. She showed rapid improvement. Pro times and partial thromboplastin times were recorded every other day. A PA and lateral chest x-ray was done, and it showed improvement from previous studies. Intakes and outputs were constantly monitored, and a Foley catheter, which had been placed prior to surgery, was maintained for three days. The patient began taking a soft diet on the third postoperative day, and by the fifth postoperative day she was back on a normal diet.

Coincidentally, a ganglion cyst was diagnosed and removed from the patient's right wrist.

The patient made a rapid recovery and was discharged on the eleventh postoperative day. She was ambulating well and her breathing was quite improved from its status on admission.

CONDITION ON DISCHARGE: Improved.

FOLLOW-UP: The patient is to follow up with Dr. Larry B. Melman two days after discharge.

DISCHARGE MEDICATIONS: Coumadin #50, 10 mg p.o. q.d., Tylenol regular strength p.r.n. pain, Azmacort inhaler, and Benadryl HCl 25 mg t.i.d. p.r.n.

DISCHARGE DIAGNOSES:
1. Asthma.
2. Pulmonary embolus, resolved.
3. Ganglion cyst, right wrist.

                              John Doe, M.D.
                              Attending Physician

JOHN DOE, M.D.
D&T: 10/12/XX | 10/13/XX | JD/mt   SMITH, HARRIET #123456-7

DISCHARGE SUMMARY

Figure 5-4 continued

MERCY MEDICAL CENTER
300 Main Street
Denver, CO 80201

DATE OF CONSULTATION: 10/06/XX

REASON FOR CONSULTATION: Dyspnea and asthma, rule out other pulmonary etiology.

CONSULTING PHYSICIAN: Lawrence B. Melman, M.D., Pulmonology

ATTENDING PHYSICIAN: John Doe, M.D.

The chart and pertinent physical findings have been reviewed. A chest x-ray was taken the morning after admission and showed a possible pulmonary embolus. Examination under fluoroscopy was performed, and it was positive for poor capillary filling and showed a plug that had been forced into a smaller one, thus obstructing the circulation. Pulmonary studies revealed the patient to have decreased lung capacity, a pulse oximetry of 88% and a high FEV to FVC ratio.

The probable diagnosis at this time is acute asthma and pulmonary embolism, causing dyspnea and poor pulmonary circulation.

RECOMMENDATIONS: My recommendation is for a pulmonary angiogram and placement of a catheter.

Thank you for your referral. I will follow this patient with you.

_____
Lawrence B. Melman, M.D.
Pulmonology Department

JOHN DOE, M.D.   SMITH, HARRIET #123456-7
Dictated by:Lawrence B. Melman, M.D.
D&T: 10/06/XX | 10/06/XX | LM/mt

CONSULTATION REPORT

Figure 5–6   Consultation Report

MERCY MEDICAL CENTER
300 Main Street
Denver, CO 80201

PREOPERATIVE DIAGNOSES: 1. Rule out pulmonary embolus.
                           2. Status post angiogram.

POSTOPERATIVE DIAGNOSES: Same.

DATE OF PROCEDURE: 10/05/XX

SURGEON: Ima Cutter, M.D.

FIRST ASSISTANT: Harry Fingers, M.D.

OPERATIONS PERFORMED: 1. Right brachial cutdown.
                       2. Pulmonary angiogram.
                       3. Placement of a Swan-Ganz catheter.

PROCEDURE: Under 2% Xylocaine local anesthesia and a Betadine prep, an incision was made over the right antecubital vein, and a #9 arterial catheter was advanced from the right antecubital area to the right pulmonary artery. Right pulmonary angiography was then done. Following this, a guide wire was placed. The arterial catheter was placed in the left main pulmonary artery, the guide wire was removed, and a left pulmonary angiogram was done. The catheter was then removed, and a Swan-Ganz catheter was advanced from the antecubital vein to the pulmonary artery. Pulmonary artery pressure was 21/8 and the pulmonary capillary wedge mean was approximately 5. The Swan-Ganz catheter was then removed.

The patient tolerated the procedure well and was returned to the recovery room in good condition.

Sponge count: Correct.

Estimated blood loss: Approximately 500 cc.

_____
Ima Cutter, M.D.
Surgeon

JOHN DOE, M.D.   SMITH, HARRIET #123456-7
Dictated by: Ima Cutter, M.D. | 10/05/XX | IC/mt
D&T: 10/05/XX | 10/05/XX | IC/mt

OPERATIVE REPORT

Figure 5–5   Operative Report

MERCY MEDICAL CENTER
300 Main Street
Denver, CO 80201

RADIOLOGY #: 23445

PA & LATERAL CHEST   Date: 10/07/XX

The pulmonary vessels are clearly outlined and are not distended.
There are not any typical signs of redistribution. A few increased
interstitial markings persist, but there are no typical acute Kerley
B-lines. There may be a little residual pleural effusion at the
costophrenic sinus and posterior gutters. Most of the pulmonary
edema and effusion has otherwise cleared. The chest is not
hyperexpanded. The thoracic vertebrae show spurring but no
compression.

IMPRESSION:
1.   No signs of elevated pulmonary venous pressure or frank failure
     at this time.
2.   Residual pleural effusion is seen in the costophrenic sinus and
     posterior gutters, either residual or recent congestive
     failure.

BILATERAL MAMMOGRAMS   Date: 10/07/XX

Bilateral xeromammograms were obtained in both the mediolateral and
craniocaudal projections. There is no previous exam for comparison.
There is slight asymmetry of the ductal tissue in the lower outer
quadrant of the right breast. There are no dominant masses, clusters
of microcalcifications or pathologic skin changes identified.

IMPRESSION: Normal bilateral mammogram.

                                        _____
                                        Renny Genray, M.D.
                                        Radiologist

JOHN DOE, M.D.   SMITH, HARRIET #123456-7
Dictated by: Renny Genray, M.D.
D&T: 10/07/XX | 10/07/XX | RG/mt

RADIOLOGY REPORT

Figure 5–8   Radiology Report

MERCY MEDICAL CENTER
300 Main Street
Denver, CO 80201

TISSUE SUBMITTED: Ganglion, right wrist.

GROSS: This is a cyst 1.6 cm in diameter. On section it contains
clear mucinous material. The cyst wall is 0.2 cm thick. The cyst is
multiloculated.

MICROSCOPIC: Microsection shows a cystic structure lined by parallel
rows of collagen. Multiple such cysts are present.

DIAGNOSIS: Ganglion, right wrist.

                                        _____
                                        Lil Culture, M.D.
                                        Pathologist

JOHN DOE, M.D.   SMITH, HARRIET #123456-7
Dictated by: Lil Culture, M.D.
D&T: 10/06/XX | 10/07/XX | LC/mt

PATHOLOGY REPORT

Figure 5–7   Pathology Report

Summary of Concepts

- Medical transcriptionists must be familiar with the basic hospital medical records formats.
- Medical transcriptionists should know the names of the basic six medical reports, the proper format for each, and the usual content of each report, including major headings and subheadings.
- Medical transcriptionists should be familiar with general formatting rules.
- Know the specific formats for each of the basic six reports.
- Be familiar with the turnaround time associated with each type of hospital report.
- Know the role turnaround time plays in a physician's admitting privileges.

Chapter 6

Medical Office Charting and Correspondence

Overview: Medical office records differ greatly from hospital medical reports. While there are six major types of reports used in hospitals, medical offices usually use only two types of medical records: the chart note and the letter. Whether a medical transcriptionist plans to work in a hospital, clinic, medical office, medical transcription service, or some other setting, he or she at some point will likely encounter medical office charting and should be acquainted with those procedures and formats.

Key Words

abstract

addendum

body of the letter

chart note

charting

checkup

codes

coding

complimentary close

copy notations

CPT-4

date

enclosure notations

envelope addressee notations

envelope postal notations

follow-up

full block style

full justified

general practitioner (GP)

HEAP format

ICD-9-CM

inside address

justified

left justified

letterhead

margins

medical office correspondence

mixed punctuation

modified block style

modified semi-block style

open punctuation

orphan

postscript	right justified
presents	salutation
preventive medicine	signature block
problem-oriented format	sign-off initials
recheck	SOAP format
reference initials	specialist
reference line	widow
return address	workup

6–A The Role of Medical Office Charting

The purpose of documenting all encounters, procedures and diagnostic assessments in a patient's chart in a medical office, or **charting,** is twofold. The first role of medical office charting is simply to provide permanent, legible written documentation of the medical record.

As you have discovered, medical offices operate quite differently from hospitals in terms of medical transcription and the documentation of medical records. In hospitals, patients usually are admitted for a short period of time or are seen, receive short-term treatment and are then referred elsewhere. Each new hospital admission is treated separately, and a new set of reports is generated for each admission.

In medical offices, however, patients usually are seen at more frequent intervals. The evaluation and treatment for each visit may be separate or linked to a previous or future visit, and the patient records in the medical office reflect this continuity. Notes from one visit may be added to a previous record, or all records may be combined.

Additionally, the turnaround time in medical offices is usually more rigid than in a hospital. Although occasionally a physician's office will have a turnaround time of 72 hours or more, because medical office patients are seen at more frequent intervals than they are in hospitals, the physician often will request a turnaround time of 24 hours or less so if the patient comes in for reevaluation all of his or her records will be posted in the chart.

The second role charting plays in the medical office is to ensure payment for the physician or medical provider. Without charting, physicians could not be paid or reimbursed by insurance companies for their services, and the medical office staff, including medical transcriptionists, in turn, could not be paid for performing their duties. Establishing and maintaining guidelines for payment policies for medical services rendered has become such a complex subspecialty of medical office administration that most medical offices have personnel or even entire departments dedicated solely to the financial aspect of health care.

The primary function medical transcription serves in ensuring that the physician is paid for his or her services is in assisting in the proper preparation of all medical records documents for coding purposes. **Coding** is transferring the narrative description of diseases, injuries, medical conditions and procedures into numerical designations. To ensure that a physician or hospital is paid, and to ensure that insurance companies are billed for the treatment of a patient, all procedures, professional medical services and diagnoses in the medical record must be assigned **codes,** universally recognized numerical indicators for a procedure, service or diagnosis. In addition to transcribing the medical record and, along with the physician, making sure it is correct and complete, medical transcriptionists are often asked to code diagnoses and procedures as they transcribe dictation, so billing and filing insurance claims will be an easier process for the medical records department.

Usually in a large medical records setting, such as a hospital, there are personnel whose primary job is to code and **abstract** (break down technical medical information into more simple terms). In smaller medical settings such as medical offices, it is often one of the combined duties of the medical transcriptionist to code and abstract medical records. Therefore, it is important that the transcriptionist be familiar with coding.

Each service or procedure a physician or other health care provider performs is documented in the record and numerically coded, and payment is based on that coding. The reference guide book that establishes the codes for a particular service or procedure is called the *Physician's Current Procedural Terminology*, Fourth Edition (**CPT-4**), which is published annually by the American Medical Association. In the hospital, all diagnoses must be coded, and the *International Classification of Diseases,* Ninth Revision, *Clinical Modification* (**ICD-9-CM**) is used for this purpose.

Although we will not explore the many facets of coding here, as stated previously, it is important that a medical transcriptionist be familiar with coding, as this could be or become part of his or her duties that augment the transcribing of medical records. For further guidelines and instruction about coding procedures, consult Delmar Publishers' *Understanding Medical Insurance,* Fourth Edition, by JoAnn Rowell.

6–B Types of Chart Notes

In terms of charting, the office note, or **chart note,** is the most frequently transcribed medical office record. There generally are three instances in which a patient would present himself or herself or be referred to a physician's office, and three corresponding types of chart notes: the **workup,** the **checkup** and the **follow-up.**

The Workup   When a patient sees a physician for the first time, he or she usually comes to the office, or **presents,** for a workup. A workup can be performed on a new patient presenting to the office for a first time or an established patient who has been to the medical office prior to the current visit. During a workup the physician investigates, or works up, the patient's problem, symptoms and complaints. A workup is made on three levels: the symptoms (the patient's perceived, or subjective, complaints), the signs (the physician's observable and verifiable, or objective, findings), and the diagnosis (the analysis of the patients condition). When dictating the workup, the physician usually will narrate the patient's history (which would include the symptoms), a physical examination (which would include the signs of the problem), an assessment (the diagnosis), and a plan (the long-term goals and direction of the treatment). Based on the number of diagnoses made or management options exercised in evaluating the patient, the intricacy of medical decision making with the workup would probably be of moderate-to-high complexity.

The Checkup   As a means of preventing disease, physicians follow a policy of preventive medicine. Often insurance companies also require that their subscribers follow a regimen of preventive medicine. **Preventive medicine** is based on a standard of consistent, regularly scheduled physician's office visits. Preventive medicine involves periodic evaluations of established patients, or checkups. In addition to providing an important means for checking on the status of patients being cared for over periods of time, checkups also are a means for checking the growth and progress of infants and children (called well-child checkups, or checks). When the physician dictates the checkup, he or she usually focuses on the physical findings, since the history is usually already known and has been explored. There often is an assessment, and a plan and brief mention of the history may be made. A checkup is not performed on a new patient, but an established one. Because the diagnosis can be either singular or multiple, but normally not very complex, and since the level of care is usually minimal or moderate, the medical decision making involved with the checkup would probably be straightforward or of low-to-moderate complexity.

The Follow-up   To monitor the status of a new patient's initial complaint(s), or to manage the continued care of an established patient, the person being treated often is scheduled to return to the physician's office for a **recheck,** or a follow-up visit. At this visit the physician reevaluates and reexamines the patient. Since the follow-up is tied to a previous report, either a workup or a checkup, when dictating this report the physician generally focuses on the assessment and plan. He or she also usually recommends a new follow-up date in this report. A brief physical exam may be included in the report, or a mention of changes in the patient's problem and some reference to the patient's history may be made. The diagnoses and level of care involved with this type of visit can range from simple to complex, therefore the type of medical decision making involved could range anywhere from low- to high-complexity.

6–C Formats for Chart Notes

Chart notes usually are done in one of two generally recognized formats: the **SOAP format** and the **HEAP format** (also known as the HPIP format). The acronyms are explained next.

The SOAP Format:
S —SUBJECTIVE (history, or what the patient tells the physician)
O—OBJECTIVE (physical exam, or what the physician discovers upon evaluation)
A—ASSESSMENT (the physician's impression of the problem, or the diagnosis)
P —PLAN (the planned course of treatment for the patient)

The HEAP Format:
H—HISTORY (equivalent to Subjective)
E —(PHYSICAL) EXAMINATION (equivalent to Objective)
A—ASSESSMENT (equivalent to Assessment or Impression)
P —PLAN (equivalent to Plan)

Often, parts of the SOAP format and HEAP format are interchanged. Always transcribe what the physician dictates, but ask if a facility or a physician would like you to keep the chart note in one particular format or another. For example, you might ask, if the physician dictates "History" followed by an "Objective" section, whether the facility wants you to leave it as such, or change "Objective" to "Physical Examination."

A third type of chart note format is the **problem-oriented format,** based on one or more specific patient problems, or complaints. The problem-oriented format begins with a statement of the first problem the patient complains of, also called a chief complaint, followed by a subjective, objective, assessment and plan regarding that problem, followed by the next problem. This problem-oriented format is often used for checkups.

6–D Types of Medical Office Correspondence

Medical office correspondence consists of letters dictated by the physician. There are two basic categories of medical doctors in private practice: the **general practitioner** (also called an internist or primary care physician [PCP]) and the **specialist,** and their correspondence varies accordingly. General practitioners, or GPs, are physicians who provide health care centered on the entire workings of the body as a whole. When GPs dictate medical office correspondence, they dictate primarily letters that introduce a patient or letters relating to a checkup or follow-up of a patient. Specialists provide health care dealing with a special system or component of the body, such as the heart (a cardiologist), the brain (a neurologist), or the sensory organs such as the ears, nose and throat (an otorhinolaryngologist). The majority of the specialist's medical office correspondence is based on the workup or follow-up of a referred patient.

Many situations arise when a physician must dictate a letter of correspondence. These include:

- letters reporting test results
- letters of introduction or referral of a patient
- letters reminding patients that they have not had certain tests or evaluations performed
- letters to patients' employers providing a medical reason for excuse from work
- letters to insurance companies requesting preauthorization for a medical procedure, review of payment made, or reevaluation of a denial of payment to an insurance company
- letters of second opinion

Physicians also dictate letters going to medical review boards, utilization review committees, hospital administration, medical staff offices and other medical personnel, letters of recommendation, and personal correspondence.

Letter Components Letters are constructed in a specific format and contain certain parts that help make them uniform, concise and clear. They usually are printed or keyed on office stationery or **letterhead,** heavy bond (weight), often textured paper that contains preprinted, typeset information about the office including names, addresses, phone and fax numbers, and the names and titles of key office personnel such as physicians, physicians' assistants, allied health professionals, and office administrators.

All letters must contain a minimal amount of information to ensure that the letter is going to whom and from whom it should, on the date it should, as well as a reference to whom or what the letter relates. The required components of a letter of medical correspondence encompass the following (each new component is placed two spaces below the previous one):

the **return address** of the physician or medical facility (or preprinted letterhead)

the **date** (the month, day and year the letter was dictated), placed at least two inches from the top margin or four spaces from the bottom line of the letterhead

the **inside address** (the name and address, including the zip code, and sometimes the phone number(s) of the party to whom the letter is addressed)

a **reference line(s)** (one or more lines with the first usually beginning with the abbreviation "RE" followed by a colon, two spaces or a tab space, and the name of the patient or the subject of the letter; subsequent lines lined up directly under the first word following the abbreviation "RE:")

the **salutation** (the greeting, such as "Dear Dr. Jones" or "To Whom It May Concern," followed by a colon for most formal or official correspondence and a comma for more personal, informal correspondence)

the **body of the letter** (the main portion, or main text, of the letter)

the **complimentary close** (the closing, such as "Sincerely" or "Very truly yours")

an underscored or blank **signature block** (three or more blank lines followed by the name and titles of the person dictating the letter, such as "Jerry Brown, M.D., F.A.C.S.")

reference/sign-off initials (the initials of the person dictating in uppercase, and the initials of the person transcribing in lowercase, separated by a colon or slash)

copy notations (the letters "pc" for photocopy or "cc" for carbon copy, often followed by a colon and the name to whom the copy is going) Many clinics and offices are now using the "pc" notation instead of the more standard but somewhat outdated "cc" to indicate that a copy needs to be sent; however, although the photocopier has replaced carbon paper in most facilities, some still prefer to use "cc" to indicate a copy being sent. Consult the facility for which you are transcribing about their preference.

enclosure notations (the word Enclosure(s) or the letters "Enc.", often followed by a colon and a description of the enclosure)

postscript(s) (additional words, lines or paragraphs added after the original completion of the letter, as an afterthought, which the dictator indicated should be an addition, or **addendum,** to the letter, expressed by using the letters "P.S." with periods separating the letters and often followed by a colon and two spaces or an indentation)

Unless otherwise indicated by a physician or facility, **margins** (space from the edge of the page) should be one inch each from the left, right and bottom margins, with at least one-half to one-inch margins from any letterhead information (whether at the top or the bottom of the page). The body of the letter should be single-spaced. The following guidelines for spacing should be used between components of the letter:

Use at least three blank lines (quadruple spacing) between the date and inside address.

Use one blank line (double spacing) between the inside address and any postal letter notations and/or reference line(s).

Use double spacing between the last reference line and the salutation.

Use single spacing throughout the body of the text of the letter.

Use double spacing between paragraphs in the body of the text.

Use double spacing between page two information at the top of page two and the continuation of the body of text.

Use double spacing between the last line of the body of text and the complimentary close.

Use at least two blank lines (triple spacing) between the complimentary close and the signature block.

Use double spacing between the signature line and the sign-off initials.

Use double spacing between the sign-off initials and any copy or enclosure notations.

Use double spacing between the end of the letter and any postscripts.

Keep the following points in mind when transcribing medical correspondence:

1. Use two-letter US state abbreviations (such as CO, WA, CA).

2. Use five- or nine-digit zip codes whenever possible.

3. Key **envelope addressee notations** (notes directed to whom the envelope is addressed, such as PERSONAL & CONFIDENTIAL, ATTN.: CLAIMS DEPARTMENT, etc.) in uppercase, three spaces below the return address block at the upper left-hand corner of the envelope. Key **envelope postal notations** (notes directed to the post office, such as VIA REGISTERED MAIL, RETURN RECEIPT REQUESTED) in uppercase, approximately one and one-half inches from the upper right-hand corner, underneath the space for postage.

Letter Styles   The appearance of a letter is crucial to a physician. Whether his or her letter is greeted by the recipient as being clear, clean and well conveyed, or whether the letter is grammatically incorrect with typographical errors and an inconsistent format, is a reflection not only on the medical transcriptionist's abilities but on the perception of the physician as well. A letter that is properly transcribed will certainly be more effective than one that is not, and incorrectly transcribed medical correspondence is not only unsatisfactory cosmetically, but its meaning may become unclear or ambiguous and could possibly invite medicolegal problems for both the physician and the medical transcriptionist. With letter writing, impression is key; therefore, it is crucial that the medical transcriptionist be knowledgeable about the various types of letter styles used for transcribing medical correspondence.

Three basic types of letter styles are used for medical office correspondence: the **full block style,** the **modified block style** and the **semi-modified block style.** With the full block style, all components of the letter such as the date, inside address, salutation, body, close, and so on, are **justified** (all text is aligned to the right, left or both margins) to one side. In this case, the entire text of the letter is **left justified** (all text is aligned to the left margin), or **full justified** (all text is placed equally between margins, with text aligned to both the left and right margins), without tabs at the beginning of paragraphs.

With the modified block style, the date, reference line(s), and complimentary close all begin at approximately the center of the page, and the remainder of the letter's components (such as the salutation and body of text) are left or full justified, without tabs at the beginning of paragraphs.

The semi-modified block style is almost identical to the modified block style, except the former uses a **right justified** date (the text of the date is aligned to the right margin) and tabs at the beginning of each paragraph.

These three styles are the ones most commonly used in medical offices; however, physicians may work with the medical transcriptionist to develop his or her own individual style, which may be a combination or variation of the three. Always consult with the physician to see if he or she prefers that letters be left justified or full justified. Also check with the dictator to see if she or he prefers **open punctuation** (no punctuation after salutations and complimentary closes) or **mixed punctuation** (the salutation is punctuated with a colon and the complimentary close is punctuated with a comma). Most physicians tend to prefer mixed punctuation, but this may vary from dictator to dictator. Additionally, always ask the physician how he or she prefers to have the date line, reference line, special mailing notations, attention lines and subject lines typed before transcribing correspondence.

Keep in mind the following points when transcribing correspondence:

1. The last word on a page should not be divided.
2. Try to avoid "widows" and "orphans" in a letter. A **widow** is one line of text at the top of a page separated from the rest of the paragraph of which it is a part; the remainder of the paragraph is located on the previous page. An **orphan** is one line of text at the bottom of a page separated from the rest of the paragraph of which it is a part; the remainder of the paragraph is located on the next page.
3. If a letter is too short to divide the last paragraph correctly, condense and complete the letter on the first page by removing spaces before and/or after the date line, putting suite numbers on the same line as the street address, and making copy and enclosure notations single-spaced instead of double-spaced.
4. The complimentary close and signature block should not stand alone on a page. Make a page break in a position that provides at least two lines of text preceding the complimentary close on the page containing the complimentary close and signature block.

6–E Specific Medical Charting and Correspondence Formats

The SOAP format for a chart note is shown in Figure 6–1. Figure 6–2 illustrates the problem-oriented format for a chart note. Figures 6–3, 6–4 and 6–5 show the three types of letter styles.

PATIENT NAME: Mary Jones
DATE: January 21, 1989

SUBJECTIVE: This is a teenager who has had a long history of recurring tonsillitis. Apparently last year she was not having too many problems, but she did as a younger child. They moved here last year, and she has been having essentially monthly episodes of tonsillitis, with a sore throat, fever, and some toxicity that usually responds to penicillin quite quickly. She is a nonsnorer and has been having problems eating solids.

OBJECTIVE: There is a 4+ right tonsil, with some deep crypts and debris. The left side is 3+ and similarly affected. There are shotty cervical nodes anteriorly. The remainder is unremarkable.

ASSESSMENT: Recurring and chronic tonsillitis, with marked hypertrophy and cryptic changes.

PLAN: We discussed the pros and cons of tonsillectomy, which I recommended to them. I let them know about the specific risks involved. Since it looks like she is acutely infected currently, I put her on amoxicillin 250 t.i.d. for 10 days. The parents will give it some thought and call back if they want to schedule it. I told them that we should put her on antibiotics a week ahead of time to try to prevent an acute flare-up.

[Space left intentionally blank for signature]

MD/mt

Figure 6–1 Chart note, SOAP format

PATENT NAME: Mary Jones
DATE: January 21, 1989

Problem 1) Tonsillitis.

SUBJECTIVE: This is a youngster who has had a long history of recurring tonsillitis. Apparently last year she was not having too many problems, but she did as a younger child. They moved here last year, and she has been having essentially monthly episodes of tonsillitis, with a sore throat, fever, and some toxicity that usually responds to penicillin quite quickly. She is a nonsnorer and has been having problems eating solids.

OBJECTIVE: There is a 4+ right tonsil, with some deep crypts and debris. The left side is 3+ and similarly affected. There are shotty cervical nodes anteriorly. The remainder is unremarkable.

ASSESSMENT: Recurring and chronic tonsillitis, with marked hypertrophy and cryptic changes.

PLAN: We discussed the pros and cons of tonsillectomy, which I recommended to them. I let them know about the specific risks involved. Since it looks like she is acutely infected currently, I put her on amoxicillin 250 t.i.d. for 10 days. The parents will give it some thought and call back if they want to schedule it. I told them that we should put her on antibiotics a week ahead of time to try to prevent an acute flare-up.

Problem 2) Right ear pain.

S: The child has been complaining of right ear pain and pressure for about a week. She has had no drainage from the ear, but the mother has noticed some possible decrease in her hearing, as she constantly asks for the television to be turned up when others are comfortable with its sound. She has a previous history of a possible left otitis media, but she has never been evaluated for tubes.

O: In the right ear the tympanic membrane is dull, beefy red and retracted. The left ear is normal. Audiogram done today shows some mild right-sided high-frequency hearing loss. The tympanogram in the right ear is type B.

A: Otitis media, right ear.

P: Augmentin 250 mg t.i.d. for two weeks. Tylenol for pain. Recheck after the medication has been completed. Consider possible consultation with an otolaryngologist for tube evaluation.

[Space left intentionally blank for signature]

JD/mt

Figure 6–2   Chart note, problem-oriented format

ASSOCIATES OF OTOLARYNGOLOGY
300 Main Street, Suite 200
Aurora, Colorado 80011

Jason Jones, M.D.   Samuel Smythe, M.D.

January 1, XXXX

John Smith, M.D.
Colorado General Practitioners, P.C.
12345 Broadway
Denver, CO 80201

via REGISTERED MAIL

RE: Mrs. Mary Jones

Dear Dr. Smith:

Thank you for referring Mrs. Jones. She is a 51-year-old woman who notes several symptoms for the past three months. She has noticed a left neck lump that has gotten slightly bigger and more tender over this period of time. She says it seemed to improve a bit while she was on Keflex, but then it came back when she stopped it. She also complains of some chronic hoarseness and cough. There has also been a lot of pressure-type headache, nasal congestion and thick, yellowish discharge. She smokes one pack per day, but was a heavier smoker earlier. She says she only drinks a few beers per week. She has also had some fever off and on. She says that she had a diagnosis of vocal cord polyps at one time several years ago.

The exam revealed a hoarse woman who was slightly nervous and just slightly above desirable weight. The tympanic membranes were clear. The audiogram and tympanogram were normal. The nasal exam shows a mild left septal deviation, with quite severe rhinitis and a lot of yellow exudate. The sinuses are nontender. The oropharynx reveals a lot of thick, yellow postnasal drip. The neck exam revealed a 1 x 1.5 cm, soft, tender mass over the left anterior cervical region, with quite prominent pulsations presumably transmitted from the deeper carotid.

Figure 6-3   The full block letter style

Letter to Dr. John Smith
RE: Mrs. Mary Jones
January 1, XXXX
Page 2

She has several symptoms that could be ominous. We went ahead with a fiberoptic exam of the larynx, and it revealed some moderate laryngitis, along with a little bit of thickening of the left anterior vocal cord with perhaps some early leukoplakia present. Our hope is that this may predominantly be from a chronic sinusitis, of which she has very strong symptoms and physical findings.

We are going to go ahead and treat her accordingly with having her finish the Keflex that she has for another four days and then start Bactrim DS b.i.d. for another 10 days. In addition, we started her on Beconase AQ, Respaire and some Fiorinal with codeine for the pain and headache. We warned her very strongly that she needs to come back for a recheck in two weeks, and, especially if the left neck lump has not improved, we will do a needle biopsy that day. We will continue to follow all the other problems until they resolve or we have to do further evaluation.

We will keep you informed of her progress.

Sincerely,

Samuel Smythe, M.D., F.A.C.S.

SS/mt

enc.: 1) Audiogram
       2) Tympanogram

pc: Jane Miller, Audiologist
       Thomas James, M.D.

Figure 6-3   continued

ASSOCIATES OF OTOLARYNGOLOGY
300 Main Street, Suite 200
Aurora, Colorado 80011

Jason Jones, M.D.   **Samuel Smythe, M.D.**

January 1, XXXX

John Smith, M.D.
Colorado General Practitioners, P.C.
12345 Broadway
Denver, CO 80201

via REGISTERED MAIL

                        RE: Mrs. Mary Jones

Dear Dr. Smith:

Thank you for referring Mrs. Jones. She is a 51-year-old woman who notes several symptoms for the past three months. She has noticed a left neck lump that has gotten slightly bigger and more tender over this period of time. She says it seemed to improve a bit while she was on Keflex, but then it came back when she stopped it. She also complains of some chronic hoarseness and cough. There has also been a lot of pressure-type headache, nasal congestion and thick, yellowish discharge. She smokes one pack per day, but was a heavier smoker earlier. She says she only drinks a few beers per week. She has also had some fever off and on. She says that she had a diagnosis of vocal cord polyps at one time several years ago.

The exam revealed a hoarse woman who was slightly nervous and just slightly above desirable weight. The tympanic membranes were clear. The audiogram and tympanogram were normal. The nasal exam shows a mild left septal deviation, with quite severe rhinitis and a lot of yellow exudate. The sinuses are nontender. The oropharynx reveals a lot of thick, yellow postnasal drip. The neck exam revealed a 1 x 1.5 cm, soft, tender mass over the left anterior cervical region, with quite prominent pulsations presumably transmitted from the deeper carotid.

Figure 6-4   The modified block letter style

To Dr. John Smith   - 2 -   January 1, XXXX
RE: Mary Jones

She has several symptoms that could be ominous. We went ahead with a fiberoptic exam of the larynx, and it revealed some moderate laryngitis, along with a little bit of thickening of the left anterior vocal cord with perhaps some early leukoplakia present. Our hope is that this may predominantly be from a chronic sinusitis, of which she has very strong symptoms and physical findings.

We are going to go ahead and treat her accordingly with having her finish the Keflex that she has for another four days and then start Bactrim DS b.i.d. for another 10 days. In addition, we started her on Beconase AQ, Respaire and some Fiorinal with codeine for the pain and headache. We warned her very strongly that she needs to come back for a recheck in two weeks, and, especially if the left neck lump has not improved, we will do a needle biopsy that day. We will continue to follow all the other problems until they resolve or we have to do further evaluation.

We will keep you informed of her progress.

                        Sincerely,

                        Samuel Smythe, M.D., F.A.C.S.

SS/mt

Enclosures: 1) Audiogram
              2) Tympanogram

pc: Jane Miller, Audiologist
       Thomas James, M.D.

Figure 6-4   continued

ASSOCIATES OF OTOLARYNGOLOGY
300 Main Street, Suite 200
Aurora, Colorado 80011

Jason Jones, M.D.   **Samuel Smythe, M.D.**

January 1, XXXX

John Smith, M.D.
Colorado General Practitioners, P.C.
12345 Broadway
Denver, CO 80201

via REGISTERED MAIL

                    RE: Mrs. Mary Jones

Dear Dr. Smith:

Thank you for referring Mrs. Jones. She is a 51-year-old woman who notes several symptoms for the past three months. She has noticed a left neck lump that has gotten slightly bigger and more tender over this period of time. She says it seemed to improve a bit while she was on Keflex, but then it came back when she stopped it. She also complains of some chronic hoarseness and cough. There has also been a lot of pressure-type headache, nasal congestion and thick, yellowish discharge. She smokes one pack per day, but was a heavier smoker earlier. She says she only drinks a few beers per week. She has also had some fever off and on. She says that she had a diagnosis of vocal cord polyps at one time several years ago.

The exam revealed a hoarse woman who was slightly nervous and just slightly above desirable weight. The tympanic membranes were clear. The audiogram and tympanogram were normal. The nasal exam shows a mild left septal deviation, with quite severe rhinitis and a lot of yellow exudate. The sinuses are nontender. The oropharynx reveals a lot of thick, yellow postnasal drip. The neck exam revealed a 1x1.5 cm, soft, tender mass over the left anterior cervical region, with quite prominent pulsations presumably transmitted from the deeper carotid.

Figure 6-5   The semi-modified block letter style

To: Dr. John Smith
RE: Mrs. Mary Jones   - 2 -   January 1, XXXX

She has several symptoms that could be ominous. We went ahead with a fiberoptic exam of the larynx, and it revealed some moderate laryngitis, along with a little bit of thickening of the left anterior vocal cord with perhaps some early leukoplakia present. Our hope is that this may predominantly be from a chronic sinusitis, of which she has very strong symptoms and physical findings.

We are going to go ahead and treat her accordingly with having her finish the Keflex that she has for another four days and then start Bactrim DS b.i.d. for another 10 days. In addition, we started her on Beconase AQ, Respaire and some Fiorinal with codeine for the pain and headache. We warned her very strongly that she needs to come back for a recheck in two weeks, and, especially if the left neck lump has not improved, we will do a needle biopsy that day. We will continue to follow all the other problems until they resolve or we have to do further evaluation.

We will keep you informed of her progress.

                    Sincerely,

                    Samuel Smythe, M.D., F.A.C.S.

SS/mt

Enclosures: 1) Audiogram
              2) Tympanogram

pc: Jane Miller, Audiologist
    Thomas James, M.D.

    P.S.: I hope you had a great time on your vacation in California. You missed some horrendous weather! Let's get together for lunch or dinner soon.

Figure 6-5   continued

Summary of Concepts

- Medical office charting is a very important part of the medical practice for documentation as well as payment purposes.
- A medical transcriptionist should become familiar with the importance and methods of medical office chart coding.
- The chart note types include the workup, checkup and follow-up, and chart note formats include the SOAP format, HEAP format and problem-oriented format.
- A medical transcriptionist should know the rules and guidelines for office note charting.
- Medical office correspondence consists of letters dictated by either a general practitioner or a specialist.
- A medical transcriptionist should know the various components and styles of medical office correspondence, and the rules and guidelines associated with each.

Chapter 7

Additional Medical Forms, Formats and Documents

Overview: In addition to the medical forms and formats with which you have already become familiar, you may as a medical transcriptionist often be asked to transcribe other types of reports, forms, and correspondence. Some of these will be explored in this chapter.

Key Words

byline	fields	merged letter
corporate minutes	font	professional corporation
curriculum vitae	form file	spreadsheets
data file	form letter	transcript
databases	memo	vocational

7–A The Form Letter

For a physician to communicate with more than one patient or colleague, with the same information in the body of text but with each piece of correspondence individually tailored to each addressee, he or she often will dictate what is called a **form letter.** A form letter is basically the shell of a letter, generated with word processing software on a computer, which contains a majority of the same information that will be sent to different persons with different addresses. Sometimes portions of the letter will contain certain areas where specific information relating to each individual addressee can be inserted, called **fields.** The addressee's name, street address, city, state, postal code, and country constitute the major fields of a form letter. Other fields can include items like titles (Dr./Mr./Ms.), gender-specific pronouns (he or she), dates, amounts, diagnoses, and other fields within the body of the text of the letter that can be customized with individual information. Form letters are used for the following as well as other types of medical correspondence:

- letters notifying patients and colleagues of an address change of a medical office
- letters used to contact patients about follow-up care or test results

- letters requesting or providing patient insurance information
- letters communicating accounts receivable or accounts payable information (such as overdue and account delinquency notices, error in payment notices, etc.)
- letters welcoming new physicians into their practices
- letters announcing new features of a physician's own practice

Usually form letters are created in the following manner. The form letter shell, or **form file,** is created and saved as a letter containing any of the various fields mentioned previously. The fields are entered individually into another file, called a **data file,** and that file is saved with another name. The information from the two files—the form file and the data file—is then brought together, or merged into a third document called a merged file, or **merged letter.** This merged letter is the final product that is sent out to each letter addressee.

Examples of a form file (Figure 7–1), a data file (Figure 7–2), and the resulting merged letter (Figure 7–3) follow.

June 3, XXXX

{Field1} {Field2} {Field3}
{Field4}
{Field5}
{Field6} {Field7}, {Field8}

Dear {Field1} {Field3}:

My optician informs me that you have not returned to our office for recommended follow-up. An abnormality was found on ocular evaluation of your eyes, and follow-up was recommended to be done in our office. Our records indicated that you have not returned for this follow-up. It is against my medical advice for you not to follow up regarding your complaint. It is not necessary that you return to our office, but we would counsel you to seek out care with an optician, ophthalmologist or other health care practitioner involved in the evaluation and treatment of the eyes in the {Field6} area. If you would like a referral to a physician, or have further questions in this regard, please contact our office at your earliest convenience.

Thank you, {Field1} {Field3}, for your attention to this matter. We look forward to hearing from you soon.

Sincerely,

Joseph Moore, M.D.

JM/mt1

Figure 7–1 A sample form file

```
{New Record}
{Field1}Mr.
{Field2}John
{Field3}Baker
{Field4}14200 Jessup Parkway
{Field5}Apt. 405
{Field6}Hot Springs
{Field7}CA
{Field8}90001
{End Record}
```

```
{New Record}
{Field1}Ms.
{Field2}Sophie
{Field3}Ledge
{Field4}333 Mann Junction Road
{Field5}
{Field6}Palm Desert Ridge
{Field7}CA
{Field8}90002
{End Record}
```

```
{New Record}
{Field1}Ms.
{Field2}Carol
{Field3}Kramer
{Field4}678 Maple Lane
{Field5}
{Field6}Big City
{Field7}CA
{Field8}90005
{End Record}
```

```
{New Record}
```

Figure 7–2   A sample data file

7–B The Curriculum Vitae

Physicians and other health care professionals sometimes must make certain career moves. Whether it involves changing the practices or hospitals with which they are associated, becoming part of a new medical cooperative, presenting a

June 3, XXXX

Mr. John Baker
14200 Jessup Parkway
Apt. 405
Hot Springs, CA 90001

Dear Mr. Baker:

My optician informs me that you have not returned to our office for recommended follow-up. An abnormality was found on ocular evaluation of your eyes, and follow-up was recommended to be done in our office. Our records indicated that you have not returned for this follow-up. It is against my medical advice for you not to follow up regarding your complaint. It is not necessary that you return to our office, but we would counsel you to seek out care with an optician, ophthalmologist or other health care practitioner involved in the evaluation and treatment of the eyes in the Hot Springs area. If you would like a referral to a physician, or have further questions in this regard, please contact our office at your earliest convenience.

Thank you, Mr. Baker, for your attention to this matter. We look forward to hearing from you soon.

Sincerely,

Joseph Moore, M.D.

JM/mt1

Figure 7–3   A sample merged letter

medical paper for review, publishing a medical paper, participating in a research study or project, or receiving continuing education in their field of expertise, physicians from time to time need to generate an extensive resume, called a **curriculum vitae.** The curriculum vitae, or CV, is a summary of a professional's personal information, education, **vocational** (work) history, and other experience, such as research, publishing and volunteer work.

The medical transcriptionist usually is charged with preparing the CV. The transcriptionist must gather the necessary information from handwritten, typewritten and oral forms, then prepare that information for presentation to the physician or others in a stepwise, chronological format. Similar to a resume, information usually is listed in descending chronological order, with the most recent experience cited first. A recent copy of the physician's CV should be kept on file, and the CV should be updated at least twice a year. (Inclusion of a physician's personal data is optional, and the decision should be left up to the physician to include or exclude it.)

Figure 7–4 depicts a sample curriculum vitae.

CURRICULUM VITAE

GENERAL INFORMATION

NAME: Michelle Harper Reese-Lopez, M.D., F.A.A.F.P., F.A.C.P.

ADDRESS: 212 Park Avenue, Suite 300
Anywhere, California 90011

PHONE: (999) 555-3434 (office)
(999) 555-5432 (fax)

OFFICES: Anytown Family Practice, P.C.
Lutheran Hospital Building
Anytown, California

Satellite office: Community Medical Center
Medical Office Park
9000 Henrietta Blvd., Suite 520
Henrietta, California 90012

PERSONAL DATA: Married: Husband's name - Ricardo   Children: 1
Date of Birth: 3/22/XX
Place of Birth: Charleston, West Virginia

EDUCATION

University of Washington School of Medicine
Seattle, Washington
Medical Doctor (M.D.) degree - June XXXX

West Virginia State College
Charleston, West Virginia
Bachelor of Science in Biochemistry (B.S.) Degree - June XXXX

POSTGRADUATE TRAINING:
Residency in Internal Medicine
University of Washington School of Medicine, Seattle, WA
July XXXX to July XXXX

Internship in General Surgery
St. Matthew's Hospital - Pacifica, CA
June XXXX to June XXXX

CONTINUING EDUCATION:
Department of Internal Medicine
University of California at Los Angeles Medical Center,
Los Angeles, CA
Subject: Laser-Assisted Uvulo-Palatoplasty
Date: September 10, XXXX
Osler Review Course
Family Medicine
March XXXX

BOARD AND LICENSURE INFORMATION

Fellow, American College of Physicians, May XXXX
Fellow, American Association of Family Practice, September XXXX
Diplomate, National Board of Medical Examiners, July XXXX
Licensee, State of California Board of Medical Examiners, July XXXX

Figure 7–4 Sample Curriculum Vitae (CV)

CURRICULUM VITAE
Michelle Harper Reese-Lopez, M.D., F.A.A.F.P., F.A.C.P.
Page Two

<u>PRESENT POSITIONS</u>

Private Practice: Anytown Family Practice, P.C.
                                   Lutheran Medical Building
                                   212 Park Avenue, Suite 300
                                   Anytown, CA 90011

Additional Positions: Member, Ad Hoc Education Committee
                                   Community Hospital Medical Group

                                   Member, Board of Directors
                                   Anytown Surgery Center

<u>HONORS AND AWARDS</u>

Graduated Summa Cum Laude,
    University of Washington School of Medicine - XXXX
Citation for High Academic Achievement - XXXX
Recipient of University of Washington
    Student Research Fellowship, XXXX

<u>PROFESSIONAL AFFILIATIONS</u>

American Academy of Internal Medicine - Family Practitioners
American Medical Association

<u>PRESENTATIONS</u>

"Escherichia coli (E. coli) and Cross-Contamination in Pacific Northwest
    Case Studies." Seattle General Hospital, May XXXX, Seattle, WA

"Hemoglobulinopathies in the Neonate." Presented at the Children's
    Hospital - Neonatal Review Course, June XXXX, Los Angeles, CA

<u>RESEARCH EXPERIENCE</u>

Efficacy of CT Scans in Patients in a Family Medicine Setting: An analysis of 100 case studies of traumatically injured and chronically ill patients.

<u>PUBLICATIONS</u>

Reese-Lopez, M.H. and Strabinski, A.A. *Statistical Research Tools in the Internal Medicine Disciplines.* Internal Medicine, XXXX; 9:402–415

<u>COMMUNITY HEALTH / VOLUNTEER EXPERIENCE</u>

Community Health Fair Volunteer, KAAA-TV Health Fair
Los Angeles, California
XXXX to present

Free Clinic Volunteer - Notre Dame Community Hospital
Jonesberg, West Virginia
June XXXX to July XXXX

Figure 7–4   continued

7–C Medical and Scientific Reports

Medical transcriptionists are sometimes asked to transcribe material other than
dictation pertaining to a particular patient. Medical seminars, presentations and

conferences, physician publications, and research work all can necessitate the need for information or data to be transcribed from oral or rough written form. This type of transcription can range in complexity from basic double space transcribing of a report to generating complex charts, graphs, **spreadsheets** (computerized numerical worksheets) and **databases** (computerized collections of data, usually text). The final document produced from this type of technical or highly specialized type of recording is often called a **transcript.**

Always consult the physician or other medical professional for whom you are transcribing regarding their preferences for format, and when no other guidelines are available use the standard report format. The standard report format includes:

- one-inch margins on all sides of the page
- left justification
- courier 12-point **font** (a type style) or similar
- centered, bold and/or underlined report title and/or subject
- centered **byline** (author identification)
- double spacing of the body of the text
- page numbering with digits at the bottom center of page

A sample of a medical transcript, transcribed in the standard report format, is illustrated in Figure 7–5.

MITRAL REGURGITATION IN THE NEONATAL PERIOD

by Xi Cho Chung, M.D. and Luigi Francelli, M.D.
Presented at the
American College of Surgeons Annual
Conference

May XXXX

Chung: Good evening, fellow colleagues. I am Xi Cho Chung, M.D., Director of the Hudson Lake Cardiac Research Group, a physician-based research consortium specializing in rodent research in the arena of mitral valvular abnormalities.

A recent research study on mitral regurgitation was conducted from May XXXX to September XXXX in 1,000 rodent population infants born with cardiac abnormalities discovered and evaluated during the immediate neonatal period. Three groups of 333 rodent neonates were studied: the first group was treated with pharmacotherapeutic modalities, the second group was treated with cardioplastic and other surgical modalities, and the third

---

Figure 7–5   A sample medical transcript

group was a control group for which no immediate treatment, other than palliative and life-sparing, treatment was rendered. Over three-quarters (75%) of the rodent neonates had developed mitral regurgitation due to papillary muscle dysfunction secondary to an anomalous left coronary artery. Of these cases, one-tenth (10%) were attributed to pulmonary artery dysfunction, one-third (33.3%) were attributed to acute myocarditis in the immediate postnatal period, one-tenth (10%) were attributed to endocardial fibroelastosis, one-quarter (25%) were attributed to endocardial cushion defect with cleft mitral valve, and one-quarter (25%) were attributed to myxomatous degeneration of the mitral valve.

I will now turn the podium over to Dr. Francelli, co-Director and co-Founder of the Hudson Lake Cardiac Research Group. He has specialized in the study of adult and infant rheumatic valvular damage and ruptured chordae tendinae in high-risk and otherwise statistically significant segments of the cardiac patient community for over 10 years. And now, Dr. Luigi Francelli. Dr. Francelli...

Francelli: Thank you, Xi. Friends, fellow cardiologists and other esteemed colleagues. Thank you for sparing a portion of your day here at this so-far quite informative and enlightening panel presentation. I would like to quickly delve into my area of expertise in this arena of study.

As you are probably quite aware, rheumatic mitral valvular regurgitation is becoming a rarer and rarer event in this day and age without mitral valve stenosis. Valvular disease that can be attributed to rheumatic heart disease is most commonly the sequelae of shortening of the valve cusps, the papillary muscles and the chordae tendinae that become affixed to the mitral valve. In this case, the regurgitation is most commonly secondary to an acute or past episode of myocardial infarction. The MI is often ascribed to ventricular aneurysm in either the absence or presence of papillary muscle fibrosis. Significant regurgitation can be evidenced by ventricular infarction occurring at the base of the papillary musculature or papillary muscle ischemia characterized by pre-regurgitant anginal episodes. Subsequently the musculature in combination with the chordae are shorter than the opposing contractile papillary muscle in conjunction with the chordae, due to a papillary muscle losing its contractility or becoming affixed to the infarcted muscle at its base.

– 2 –

Figure 7–5 continued

7–D Medical Office Business Formats and Documents

It is often the responsibility of the medical transcriptionist to prepare specialized medical office documentation that, again, is not necessarily patient oriented. This documentation often follows a business-type format.

The interoffice memorandum, or **memo,** documents communications between office staff, usually generated by administration and addressed to one or more employees. The memo serves to maintain a good flow of office communications.

A second type of medical office documentation with which a medical transcriptionist should be familiar is the transcription of **corporate minutes.** Corporate minutes are recorded documentations of a corporate meeting, usually handwritten or dictated at the time of the meeting. Since most medical practices are specialized types of corporations, called **professional corporations,** or P.C.s, corporate meetings are held at least quarterly, and minutes must be generated and kept on file in the corporate records for each meeting. One of the physicians of the corporation is usually the secretary and is responsible for preparing and recording the minutes.

Examples of a memo and corporate minutes are shown in Figures 7-6 and 7-7.

MEMO

TO: Mary Jacobs and Milicent Harper, Staff Audiologists

FROM: George Parker, Office Administrator *GP*

DATE: May 12, XXXX

RE: Audiology Conference in Houston, Texas

This communication is to notify you that you are eligible to attend the National Audiometric Association Audiology Conference to be held in Houston, Texas, during the week of July 22–29, XXXX. Arrangements have been made with Worldglobe Travel for hotel accommodations at the Vacation Inn Hotel and Conference Center in Houston, with rental of one midsize car through Economocar. Please contact me with your flight request, and I will try to coordinate your travel plans. You are eligible for full compensation for all pertinent expenses related to the conference, including meals and other out-of-pocket expenses.

If you have any further questions, please stop by my office to discuss the details of the conference in greater detail.

GP/mt

pc: Marta Grinkov, M.D.

Figure 7–6   The interoffice memorandum format

DAIRYLAND PODIATRY, P.C.
CORPORATE MINUTES
September 30, XXXX

The quarterly meeting of Dairyland Podiatry, P.C., was held on September 11, 1996, at Barney's Restaurant and Grill. The meeting was called to order by the Corporate President, Merlin Monroe. In attendance were Merlin Monroe, M.D., D.P., President, Jules Gunther, D.P., and Julie Gentry, Office Administrator.

Resolutions

1)   WHEREAS it is deemed in the best interest of the Corporation to appoint Corporate counsel, it is therefore
RESOLVED that Kramer, Kramer and Long, Attorneys at Law, be retained as Corporate Counselor.

2)   WHEREAS it is deemed in the best interest of the Corporation to lease company vehicles from time to time for the business use of its officers and employees, and
WHEREAS the Corporation has leased a XXXX Carlisle Courier and a XXXX Monata Mover to be used by the Corporation officers while conducting Corporation business,
RESOLVED that the leases by the Corporation to be used in the Corporation's business is ratified, approved and affirmed.

New Business
1)   Discussion of office lease space and planning for future needs.
2)   Discussion of insurance contracts.
3)   Discussion of quarterly bonus for doctors and staff.

RATIFICATION

IT IS RESOLVED that all acts of the officers and directors of the Corporation and the general conduct of the business of the Corporation during the period beginning June 1, XXXX, and ending September 30, XXXX, are approved, ratified and adopted.

(continued)

Figure 7–7   Corporate minutes

DAIRYLAND PODIATRY, P.C.
C O R P O R A T E   M I N U T E S
September 30, XXXX   page 2

EFFECT OF CONSENT

This consent of the Board of Directors and Shareholders of the Corporation may be certified by any proper officer of the Corporation as having been unanimously adopted by vote of the Board of Directors and Shareholders of the Corporation on the 30th day of September, XXXX.

In Witness Whereof, the undersigned Directors and Shareholders have evidenced their approval of the above proceedings as of the date last above mentioned.

Signed: _____
                    Merlin M. Monroe, M.D., D.P.

Signed: _____
                    Jules A. Gunter, D.P.

MMM/mt

Figure 7–7   continued

Summary of Concepts

- A form letter is a letter that combines, or merges, information from a data file with information in a form file to produce a merged letter that can contain the same information in a letter or form sent to several addressees at one time.
- Periodically, physicians generate an extensive resume, called a curriculum vitae, which is a summary of the professional's education, vocational history, publications, and other pertinent professional experience.
- Medical transcriptionists are sometimes asked to transcribe material other than dictation pertaining to a particular patient. These types of documents include medical reports, transcripts, memos and corporate minutes.

Part Three

Medical Transcription Mechanics

Chapter 8

Word Usage

Overview: Medical transcriptionists must not only be well skilled in the formats involved in medical transcription, they must be very highly skilled in the literary aspects of language. After all, transcriptionists transform oral language into written language, and to do so most effectively must have a full command of spelling, punctuation and grammar, and usage in a variety of situations. A competent transcriptionist will recognize that "there" and "their" sound alike, but have different meanings, or that "pyelography" and "cystography" are synonyms. Once the medical transcriptionist is familiar with phonetics, etymology, acronyms, homonyms, synonyms and antonyms, he or she will be able to correctly edit unclear or imprecise dictation into comprehensible and accurate word-processed transcription.

Key Words

acronym	phoneme	root
antonym	phonetic group	suffix
combining form	phonetics	syllables
etymology	prefix	synonym
homonym		

8–A Phonetics and Phonemes

The study of the categorization of words according to their sounds is called **phonetics.** Phonetics can assist the medical transcriptionist in the pronunciation of the spoken word and can provide clues regarding the spelling of a word. A **phoneme** is the smallest unit of phonetics. A phoneme distinguishes one sound from another. Many phonemes together constitute a **phonetic group,** and many phonetic groups together comprise a word.

To begin to understand just how a medical transcriptionist transforms simple or complex oral expressions of phonemes and phonetics into written medical words, a thorough understanding of phonetics must be accomplished. To begin our study of phonetics, let us first look at the various phonemes that go into basic word sounds.

1. Long (Hard) Vowel Sound Phonemes. (Bold letters denote stressed syllable(s), italics denote secondary stressed syllables, and capitalized letters denote an entire phonetic sound.)

Phoneme	Word Example	Phonetic Pronunciation
Long "A" sounds:		
AY	headache	**hed**-AYk
AY	abeyance	ah-**bAY**-ehns
AY	kaolin	**kAY**-oh-lihn
Long "E" sounds		
EE	glioma	glEE-**oh**-mah
EE	peroneal	*pehr*-oh-**nEE**-al
EE	lithotomy	lith-**ot**-oh-mEE
Long "I" sounds:		
I/Y	islet	**I**-let
I/Y	myasthenia	*mY*-ahs-**thee**-nee-ah
I/Y	meiosis	mY-**oh**-sis
Long "O" sounds		
O/OH	ovum	**O**-vuhm
O/OH	peau d'orange	**pOH**-dOH-*ranj*
O/OH	vertigo	**vehr**-tih-gO
Long "U" sounds:		
YOO	uvula	**YOO**v-yah-luh
YOO	cornua	**corn**-YOO-uh
YOO	ageusia	ah-**gYOO**-see-ah

2. Short (Soft) Vowel Sound Phonemes.   (Bold letters denote stressed syllable(s), italics denote secondary stressed syllables, and capitalized letters denote an entire phonetic sound.)

Phoneme	Word Example	Phonetic Pronunciation
Soft "A" sounds:		
AH/A	action	**Ack**-shun
AH/A	compassion	cuhm-**pAH**-shun
Soft "E" sounds:		
EH/E	estrogen	**Es**-troh-gEn
EH/E	competent	**kohhm**-pEH-tEnt
Soft "I" sounds:		
IH/I/EE	itch	**Ich**
IH/I/EE	minimal	**mIH**-nIH-*mul*
IH/I/EE	antianemic	*an*-tEE-ah-**nee**-mIk
Soft "O" sounds		
OHH/O	ostracize	**Oss**-trah-syz
OHH/O	antibiotic	*an*-tih-by-**OHH**-tik
OO	loose	**lOO**s
OO	igloo	**ig**-lOO

Phoneme	Word Example	Phonetic Pronunciation
Soft "U" sounds:		
UH/U	utter	**UH**-tehr
UH/U	uterus	**yoo**-tehr-Us

3. Keys to Pronunciation and Locating the Correct Spelling of Words.

Vowels:

If the word contains this phoneme:	**Try these spellings:**
A/AY . . . (as in "apex")	a . . . , ae . . . , ai . . . , ao . . . , ay . . . , ei . . . , eh . . . , et . . . , ey . . . (Examples: ameliorate, aerodigestive, capsaisin, aortic, decay, weigh, Fehling's solution, bouquet, grey)
A/AH . . . (as in "apple")	a . . . , aa . . . , ah . . . (Examples: atom, graafian, Fahrenheit)
E/EE . . . (as in "edict")	e . . . , ea . . . , ee . . . , ei . . . , eo . . . , ae . . . , ie . . . , i . . . , oe . . . , y . . . (Examples: equivalent, each, eel, receive, people, fasciae, Siemens, Karposi, oesophagostomiasis, thyroidectomy)
E/EH . . . (as in "elephant")	e . . . , ea . . . , eh . . . , ie . . . , oe . . . , ue . . . (Examples: pendular, head, Behcet's syndrome, patient, roetgen, guest)
I/Y . . . (as in "ice")	i . . . , y . . . , ie . . . , ei . . . , ey . . . , ai . . . , ay . . . , igh . . . (Examples: mind, myopathy, beautified, height, Frey's syndrome, guaiac, bayou, thigh)
I/IH . . . (as in "impulse")	i . . . , e . . . , ei . . . , y . . . (Examples: inferior, pendular, ageism, myringitis)
O/OH . . . (as in "open")	o . . . , oa . . . , oh . . . , oo . . . , eau(x) . . . (Examples: olfactory, coat, Crohn's disease, oospore, rouleau [rouleaux—plural])
O/OHH . . . (as in "often")	o . . . , ou . . . , a . . . , au . . . , aw . . . (Examples: somnambulist, cough, spa, cautery, thaw)
U/OO . . . (as in "spoon")	oo . . . , u . . . , eu . . . , ou . . . , oe . . . , ue . . . (Examples: balloon, tubectomy, leukemia, douche, canoe, construe)
U/YOO . . . (as in "amuse")	u . . . , ue . . . , eu . . . , ew . . . , hu . . . , yu . . . (Examples: uvula, Mueller, eunuch, pewter, Hugier's Yutopar)
U/UH . . . (as in "upset")	u . . . , a . . . , o . . . (Examples: uncinate, canal, other)

Consonants:

**If a portion of a word begins
with this sound:**   **That part could begin with these letters:**

B . . .   b . . . , p . . . , v . . .
hard C . . . (as in "cake")   c . . . , ch . . . , qu . . . , k . . . , g . . .
soft C . . . (as in "cement")   c . . . , s . . . , ps . . . , z . . .
D . . .   d . . . , t . . .
F . . .   f . . . , ph . . . , pf . . . , v . . . , p . . . , th . . .
hard G . . . (as in "gamble")   g . . . , c . . . , k . . . , qu . . .
soft G . . . (as in "giraffe")   g . . . , j . . . , ch . . .
hard H . . . (as in "hand")   h . . . , wh . . . , i . . .
soft H . . . (as in "an historical")   h . . . , a . . . , e . . . , i . . . , o . . . , u . . . , y . . .
J . . .   j . . . , g . . . , ch . . .
K . . .   k . . . , c . . . , ch . . . , qu . . . , g . . .
L . . .   l . . .
M . . .   m . . . , mn . . . , n . . . , nm . . .
N . . .   n . . . , gn . . . , kn . . . , m . . . , mn . . . , pn . . .
P . . .   p . . . , b . . . , f . . . , v . . .
Q . . .   qu . . . , kw . . . , cu . . . , gu . . .
R . . .   r . . . , rh . . .
S . . .   s . . . , c . . . , ps . . . , z . . .
T . . .   t . . . , pt . . . , d . . . , ch . . .
V . . .   v . . . , f . . . , ph . . . , pf . . . , p . . . , b . . .
hard W . . . (as in "wall")   w . . . , wh . . .
soft W . . . (as in "who")   wh . . . , h . . .
X . . .   x . . . , z . . . , cy . . . , s . . . , ech . . . , ex . . .
Y . . .   y . . . , l . . . , u . . .
Z . . .   z . . . , x . . . , s . . . , c . . . , ps . . .

How to use the keys to pronunciation for the preceding pages:

1. Break down the word you are hearing into sounds and **syllables** (stressed word parts).
2. Try looking up all possible word beginnings, middles, and endings, using the previously mentioned sounds. The most common spelling for each sound is the first letter(s) written, and the last letter written is the least common spelling for the sound.
3. Example: dictated word: "*SOO*-doh-tehr-IHHG-ee-uhm". If you are unsure of the spelling, you would begin by looking under the possibilities for "S," which are "s . . . ", "c . . . ", "ps . . . ", "z . . . ", then combine the second sound "OO", which are "o . . . ", "oo . . . ", "u . . . ", "eu . . . ", the third sound, "D", which are "d . . . ", "t . . . ", and so on.

     You would, therefore, begin looking under words beginning with the letter "S". First you would consider words beginning in "so . . . ", but you would not find any words beginning in "so . . . " sounding like "SOO" followed by a "doh" sound. You would then look under "su . . . ", and you would find some words beginning in "sudo . . . " sounding like "SOO" followed by a "doh" sound, but none of them with the additional sounds of "tehr", "IHHG", "ee", or "uhm". You would therefore next look under "seu", and follow the same process that you did with "so"; through this process, you would not find the correct word.

After exhausting the "s . . ." possibilities, you would next start looking under words beginning with the letter "C". You would soon realize that words beginning with "co . . .", "coo . . .", and "cu . . .", would all have a hard "c" sound when followed by a vowel, and you would not pursue looking in that direction. You might look under "ceu . . ." thinking that this combination of letters could have a soft "c" sound, but you would not have any luck finding the correct word.

You would next look under the letter combination of "ps", which also forms the letter "S" sound. You would perhaps begin looking under "pso . . .", "psu . . .", and finally "pseu . . .", where you would see a word with the phonation similar to "*SOO*-doh-tehr-IHHG-ee-uhm", spelled "pseudopterygium."

8–B Etymology

Etymology is the study of word origins. Etymology helps break down words by the meaning and origin of their parts. When medical transcriptionists use etymologic tools, they are aided by the meanings of the roots, prefixes and suffixes.

Roots are the basic components of words. A root is the most simple element of a word from which its meaning can be derived. A root can be changed both in meaning and phonetically by the addition of either a beginning word portion (called a **prefix**) or an ending word portion (called a **suffix**).

A root combined with a slash (/) and the letter "o" constitutes what is called the **combining form.** With combining forms, words used in a medical context can form other words. In the example "chrom/o/meter", the definition of the word would come from the combining form "chrom/o", which means color, with the suffix "-meter" added to the root. The word now takes on a new meaning— "instrument that measures color." Another word, "achromic", can be formed with the addition of both a prefix (a-) and a suffix (-ic) to form a word meaning characterized by being without color. Most medical words are the combination of one or more root words, prefixes and/or suffixes.

The medical transcriptionist should become familiar with the meanings of the most common prefixes used in medical terminology: *a-, ab-, ad-, ante-, anti-, bi-, brady-, con-, dys-, ecto-, endo-, epi-, extra-, hyper-, hypo-, in-, inter-, intra-, mal-, neo-, para-, peri-, post-, pre-, pro-, re-, retro-, sub-, sym-, syn-, tachy-, trim, ultra-,* and *uni-.* He or she also should become familiar with the meanings of the most common suffixes used in medical terminology: *-algia, -cele, -cision, -cyte, -ectomy, -emia, -gram, -graph, -ia, -iac, -iasis, -ic, -itis, -lith, -logy, -lysis, -metry, -mortem, -oma, -osis, -partum, -pathy, -philia, -phobia, -plasm, -plasty, -plegia, -pnea, -rrhea, -scopy, -stomy, -thesis, -tomy, -trophy,* and *-uria.*

When a common prefix (such as "anti-") and common suffix (such as "-ic") is added to a common root form (such as "bi/o" or metr/o"), you will find a common medical word, such as "antibiotic". Most medical words are formed in this manner. Sometimes it is easier to understand the entire meaning of a word by breaking down its various parts.

8-C Acronyms

Acronyms are words comprised of the first letters of a series of words in a phrase, which are sometimes pronounced as a word. Try to use the series of words when possible, instead of the acronyms, unless it is the physician's or the hospital's personal style, or it is a widely accepted form. Some common acronyms (an asterisk preceding the acronym denotes that the acronym is acceptable in most transcription on first reference) follow:

*AIDS—acquired immune deficiency syndrome
CABG—coronary artery bypass graft
ECHO—enteric cytopathic human orphan (virus)
*ECoG—electrocochleography
EOMI—extraocular movements intact
*FANA—fluorescent antinuclear antibody
*HEENT—head, ears, eyes, nose and throat
MAST—military antishock treatment
PERRLA—pupils equal, round and reactive to light and accommodation
*REM—rapid eye movement
*SIDS—sudden infant death syndrome
SOAP—subjective, objective, assessment, plan
*TENS—transcutaneous electrical nerve stimulation

Some acronyms have become so common that they are now acceptable words. When acronyms become acceptable words, they are written lowercase. Some examples follow:

laser (light amplification by stimulated emission of radiation)
radar (radio detecting and ranging)
dopa (dihydroxyphenylalanine)
scuba (self-contained underwater breathing apparatus)
snafu (situation normal, all fouled up)

8-D Homonyms

Homonyms are words that sound or are pronounced alike, but are different in meaning. Medical transcriptionists often confuse homonyms, such as "the patient is to follow 'oral' hygiene for his cerumen problem." Upon closer review, it is evident that the word "oral" is a homonym for the word "aural", meaning "pertaining to the ear", and the latter word is the one and only correct word to use in this sentence. Therefore, a medical transcriptionist must always be on the lookout for confusing homonyms in dictation.

Some examples of homonyms follow:

aural (pertaining to the ears) vs. **oral** (pertaining to the mouth)
coarse (thick) vs. **course** (a path or regimen)

complement (that which completes) vs. **compliment** (praise)
ileum (intestine) vs. **ilium** (hip bone)
principal (primary) vs. **principle** (a rule or law)
their (belonging to them) vs. **there** (a place away from here)

8–E Synonyms

Synonyms are words that have the same meaning. The medical transcriptionist should become familiar with synonyms, because dictators sometimes ask that a different medical synonym be used in the transcription if they are repeating a word.

Some examples of synonyms follow:

good = just = pure = kind = generous
difficult = complex = laborious = hard = strenuous
sound = audibility = acoustics = sonification = bruit
disease = illness = sickness = ailment = malady

8–F Antonyms

Antonyms are words that have opposite meanings. Sometimes physicians mistakenly give an antonym for a word they are dictating. The medical transcriptionist must be familiar with antonyms and must be prepared to use the correct word at all times.

Some examples of antonyms follow:

hypertension (high blood pressure) vs. **hypotension** (low blood pressure)
principal (main) vs. **secondary** (less important)
macroscopic (visible to the naked eye) vs. **microscopic** (visible only with enlargement)
abduct (to flex away from) vs. **adduct** (to flex toward)
bradycardia (slow pulse rate) vs. **tachycardia** (fast pulse rate)

Summary of Concepts

- Phonetics can assist the medical transcriptionist in the pronunciation of the spoken word.
- Phonemes can assist the medical transcriptionist in figuring out what a dictator is saying, or can provide clues regarding the spelling of a word.
- Two important keys that will assist the medical transcriptionist in spelling a word are: 1) break down the word that is heard into sounds and syllables, and 2) try to look up all possible word beginnings, middles and endings, using its sounds.
- The most common spelling for each sound is the first letter(s) written, and the last letter written is the least common spelling for the sound.
- Etymology helps break down words by the meaning and origin of their parts.

- When medical transcriptionists use etymologic tools, they are aided by the meanings of the roots, prefixes, and suffixes.
- The medical transcriptionist should try to use the series of words an acronym stands for instead of its letters when possible, unless it opposes the physician's or hospital's personal style or the acronym is a widely accepted form.
- A medical transcriptionist must always be on the lookout for confusing homonyms in dictation.
- A medical transcriptionist should be familiar with synonyms, because dictators sometimes ask for a different medical synonym in the transcription if they are repeating a word.
- Sometimes physicians mistakenly provide an antonym for a word they are dictating; therefore, a medical transcriptionist must be familiar with antonyms and must be prepared to use the correct word at all times.

Chapter 9

Sentence Grammar

Overview: A medical transcriptionist should have a thorough command of the English language, and must possess excellent grammatical skills. A transcriptionist should understand in detail parts of speech and sentence structure, including nouns, verbs, adverbs, adjectives, subjects, objects, predicates, clauses, articles, conjunctions, interjections and prepositions. This chapter may be used as a refresher course in grammar and as a reference when transcribing situations may require that a grammar text be consulted.

Key Words

abstract nouns

adjectives

adverbs

article

clause

collective nouns

common nouns

concrete nouns

conjunction

coordinating conjunctions

demonstrative pronouns

direct objects

future tense

gerunds

indefinite pronouns

indirect objects

infinitive (verb form)

intensive pronouns

intransitive verbs

irregular verbs

nonrestrictive clauses

nouns

objective case

objects

past participle

past tense

personal pronouns

phrase

possessive case

predicates

prepositional phrase

prepositions

present participle

pronouns

proper nouns	subjects
reflexive pronouns	transitive verbs
regular verbs	verbal nouns
relative pronouns	verbal phrase
restrictive clauses	verbs
subjective case	

9-A Grammar Basics

All sentences are comprised of simple word parts. Often, when dictating medical records, physicians and other dictators overlook basic parts of speech and incorrectly use sentence grammar. Therefore, it is important for a medical transcriptionist to be especially proficient in sentence grammar. He or she must not only know the correct medical word or word form to use, but must be able to use the correct English word or word form. A medical transcriptionist must be able to quickly and efficiently transform the spoken word into the written word.

The basic parts of speech will be discussed next.

9-B Nouns, Subjects and Objects

Nouns

Nouns are words that refer to persons, places, things, ideas or qualities. Nouns are used more frequently than any other part of speech, and many sentences contain more than one noun. Nouns are classified as proper, common, concrete, abstract, collective and verbal. Be sure to know when to capitalize nouns used in medical dictation.

1. **Proper nouns** are formal names of persons, place and things, and they are capitalized.
   Examples: Bob went to Mercy Hospital.
   I found out that Dr. Miller attended school in Detroit, Michigan.
   Chairman Roger Rose attended the Parkinson's Disease Symposium.

2. **Common nouns** are more casual names and words, and they are not capitalized.
   Examples: The mother took her child to the emergency room.
   She took the gurney into the surgical area.
   The physician worked with the psychologist.

3. **Concrete nouns** are common nouns that refer to things perceived through the physical senses of sight, sound, smell, taste and touch.
   Examples: The physician noted the odor of ethanol on the patient's breath.

> A purulent <u>drainage</u> was emanating from the <u>wound</u>.
> She palpated a <u>sialolith</u> in the <u>gland</u>.

4. **Abstract nouns** are words that refer to things that cannot be perceived through the physical senses, such as ideas or qualities.

> *Examples:*   The guest speaker had an enlightened <u>philosophy</u>.
> Her <u>theories</u> broke <u>convention</u>.
> The surgeon proposed electrocautery as a <u>solution</u> to the <u>problem</u>.

5. **Collective nouns** are words that identify groups. Although collective nouns can express more than one person or thing, they usually are regarded as singular words.

> *Examples:*   A <u>committee</u> selects medical school candidates.
> The patient had suffered a sting after being surrounded by a <u>swarm</u> of bees.
> His <u>family</u> consented to the risks of the procedure.

6. **Verbal nouns** are words that begin with a verb and end in "-ing" but function as nouns. Verbal nouns also are called **gerunds.**

> *Examples:*   <u>Editing</u> is an important part of transcription.
> The nursing student said that <u>studying</u> had always been difficult for him.
> <u>Cleaning</u> and <u>dressing</u> a drain site daily can inhibit contamination.

Subjects

Subjects are words—usually nouns or a group of words including nouns—that are the topic(s) of a sentence. The subject of a sentence can consist of words that name something, someplace or someone, plus other words such as modifiers, conjunctions and prepositions.

> *Examples*:   The <u>hemostat</u> was within the surgeon's reach.
> <u>He</u> gave the patient an injection.
> The <u>result</u> of lack of vitamin C can be scurvy.

Objects

Objects are words—usually nouns or a group of words including nouns—that receive the action of a verb. They are different from the subject of the sentence in that the *subject performs an action* while an action is *performed upon or by an object.* There are **direct objects,** which complete the meaning of the main verb of a sentence or clause, and **indirect objects,** which identify to or for whom the direct object is performed.

> *Examples:*   The medical transcription student studied <u>pharmacology</u>. (direct object)
> He preferred <u>the well-trained nurse</u>. (direct object)
> The technician gave the Bovie unit to <u>the first assistant</u>. (indirect object)
> The residents asked <u>the professor</u> a question. (indirect object)

9–C Pronouns

Pronouns are simply words that substitute for nouns and function in sentences like nouns. Pronouns can be classified as personal, demonstrative, relative, interrogative, reflexive, intensive and indefinite. There are three cases of pronouns: the **subjective case** (where the pronoun is the subject in a sentence), the **possessive case** (where the pronoun shows possession or ownership), and the **objective case** (where the pronoun is the object in a sentence). Pronouns can be further identified as being singular or plural, and as being first person, second person or third person (see the figures that follow).

It is especially important for transcriptionists to become familiar with classifications and cases of pronouns, because dictators often confuse the cases (switching the subjective with the objective case, and vice versa), fail to use the correct pronoun, and so on. The following information can be used as a guide:

1. **Personal pronouns** are noun substitutes that refer to a particular person or group of people. Personal pronouns include the words *I, you, he, she, it, we, you, they,* and so on.

   Examples: I (subjective personal pronoun) gave his (possessive personal pronoun) CV to her (objective personal pronoun).

   They (subjective personal pronoun) showed our (possessive personal pronoun) transcription exercises to you (objective personal pronoun).

   The patient will make an appointment with (prepositional phrase) you or me (objective pronouns).

   (Special note: If you are in doubt about which personal pronoun to use, refer to Figure 9–1. If the word the pronoun replaces is a subject, regardless of where it occurs in a sentence, use the subjective pronoun. If the word the pronoun replaces is an object, regardless of where it occurs in a sentence, use the objective pronoun. Physicians often use "I" in place of an objective pronoun [*me,* or *myself*]. Remember: *prepositional phrases take objective pronouns.*)

	Subjective	Possessive	Objective
Singular			
1st person	I	my, mine	me
2nd person	you	your, yours	you
3rd person	he, she, it	his, her(s), its	him, her, it
Plural			
1st person	we	our, ours	us
2nd person	you	your, yours	you
3rd person	they	their, theirs	them

Figure 9–1 Personal pronouns

	Subjective	Objective
Singular	this/that	this/that
Plural	these/those	these/those

Figure 9–2 Demonstrative pronouns

2. **Demonstrative pronouns** are noun substitutes that identify nouns and are always either subjective or objective in case. Demonstrative pronouns include the words *this, that, these* and *those* (see Figure 9–2).

   Examples: This has a higher frequency of infection than that.
   These are more highly trained than those.

3. **Relative pronouns** link a clause to another pronoun or noun. Interrogative pronouns are noun substitutes that introduce questions. Relative pronouns include the words *who, which* and *that*. Interrogative pronouns include the words *who, which* and *what* (see Figure 9–3).

   Examples: They were the physicists who traveled from Atlanta.
   (reflexive pronouns)
   Now tell me, which x-ray film showed the oblique view?
   (interrogative pronoun)

4. **Reflexive pronouns** are noun substitutes that show that the subject of the sentence also receives the action of the verb. **Intensive pronouns** are noun substitutes that stress a noun or another pronoun.

   Examples: They have no one to blame but themselves. (reflexive)
   I myself saw the physician question the patient. (intensive)

   (Special note: Reflexive/intensive pronouns either: 1) emphasize a noun or other pronoun, or 2) indicate that the subject of the sentence also receives the action of the main verb; therefore, every time a reflexive or intensive pronoun is included, make sure there is an additional subject or pronoun in the sentence. See Figure 9–4.)

	Subjective	Possessive	Objective
Singular or Plural			
3rd person	who	whose	whom
	whoever	———	whomever
	which, that, what	———	which, that, what

Figure 9–3 Relative pronouns

	Objective
Singular	
1st person	**myself**
2nd person	**yourself**
3rd person	**herself, himself, itself**
Plural	
1st person	**ourselves**
2nd person	**yourselves**
3rd person	**themselves**

Figure 9–4   Reflexive/intensive pronouns

5. **Indefinite pronouns** are special pronouns that do not substitute for a specific noun but refer to one or a group of unknown, or indefinite, nouns. See Figure 9–5 for a complete list of indefinite pronouns.

Some rules for indefinite pronouns:

a. Indefinite pronouns always take singular pronouns:

> *Example:*   Everybody prefers his own computer equipment.
>
>   ↕   ↕
>
>   indefinite   singular
>
>   pronoun   pronoun

b. Indefinite pronouns usually take a singular verb, but the indefinite pronouns *all*, *any*, *none*, and *some* may take a plural verb. The indefinite pronouns *all*, *any*, *none*, and *some* may be either singular or plural in their meanings, and the verb used with each depends on its meaning, singular or plural, within

all	each	neither	one
any	either	nobody	some
anybody	everybody	none	somebody
anyone	everyone	no one	someone
anything	everything	nothing	something

Figure 9–5   Indefinite pronouns

a particular sentence. If the indefinite pronoun has a singular meaning, it takes a singular verb (e.g., "some" is plural in *"Some Like it Hot,"* and "some" is singular in "some goes in this tube, and some in the other"), and vice versa.

Examples: All patients go to admissions before having day surgery.

         ↕   ↕

    indefinite   plural
    pronoun   verb

None of the insurance premium covers the cost of

    ↕   ↕   infertility tests.

    indefinite   singular
    pronoun   verb

9–D Verbs and Verb Forms

Verbs are words that express actions, happenings or states of being. Some sentences contain one word that serves as a verb, while other sentences contain more than one word that serves as a verb. Multiple-word verbs contain helping verbs, or words besides the main verb that show changes in time or tense. Some groups of verbs can go together to express one action and become verb clauses.

Examples: The operation occurred the day after the holiday.
The sinusitis was camouflaged by rhinitis. ("was" is a helping verb)
Many expert transcriptionists aspire to become physicians. ("aspire to become" is a verb clause)

Verb Forms and Types

1. There are five major verb forms: the infinitive or plain form, the present participle form, the past tense form, the past participle form, and the future tense form. The **infinitive,** or plain form, of a verb is the word that will be found in the dictionary with the word *to* added before it (e.g., *to begin*). The **present participle** form of a verb is created by adding "-ing" to the infinitive of the verb (e.g., *working*). The **past tense** form of a verb indicates that the action of the verb happened in the past (e.g., *smoked*). The endings "-d" and "-ed" usually indicate that the verb is in the past tense (see #2 for exceptions). The **past participle** form is the verb form that would be used with "has", "have" or "had" (e.g., have *gone*); the form that takes a form of "be" in the passive voice (e.g., was *done*); or the form that is used by itself to modify nouns and pronouns (e.g., *blocked* artery). The **future tense** form of a verb indicate that the action of the verb will happen at some time in the future (e.g., *will operate*). The helping verbs "will" or "shall" before the plain form of the verb indicate the future tense.

    Examples: I transcribe medical records. (plain or infinitive form)
    We like transcribing medical records. (present participle form)

I <u>transcribed</u> medical records yesterday. (past tense form)

<u>Transcribed</u> reports need to be posted every evening. (past participle form)

I <u>will transcribe</u> 50 medical records tomorrow. (future tense)

2. There are two types of verbs, regular and irregular. **Regular verbs** such as "stop", "live" and "collect" take standard endings when changing tense; **irregular verbs** such as "begin", "build" and "come" take nonstandard endings or become different words entirely when changing tense. To show a change in time to the past tense for regular verbs, simply add a "d" or an "-ed" ending. To show a change in time to the past (the past tense or the past participle forms of the verb) for irregular verbs, additional changes must be made. It is important for the medical transcriptionist to become familiar with irregular verb forms, because dictators sometimes use the wrong irregular verb or verb form.

   Examples: I <u>forgot</u> the answer. (irregular past tense)

   He <u>had chosen</u> the five surgical candidates. (irregular past participle)

Figure 9–6 on page 106 provides a list of the past tenses and past participles of common irregular verbs.

Predicates

Predicates are words—usually verbs or groups of words containing verbs—that describe actions, happenings or states of being.

   Examples: The patient <u>was examined</u> under anesthesia.

   The symposium <u>featured</u> several expert proctologists.

   Operations <u>take</u> time.

9–E Word Modifiers and Determiners

Adjectives

Adjectives are words that describe or modify nouns or pronouns. An adjective can be a single word or word group that modifies. Note: Medical terms that are adjectives often end in *-ic, -al, -able, -ible,* or *-ian,* and compound adjectives often have a delineating word as a prefix such as *well-, post-, right-, left-, low-,* and so on.

   Examples: The <u>leukorrheic</u> hemorrhage was a complication of the procedure.

   The infant was <u>well nourished</u>.

   Her <u>soft-spoken</u> manner was much appreciated.

Adverbs

Adverbs are words that describe or modify verbs, adjectives and other adverbs. Note: Very few medical terms are adverbs, but many terms that are usually adjectives can become adverbs when "-ly" is added to the end of the word.

   Examples: The drug education pamphlet was <u>carefully</u> worded.

   The abscess was draining <u>profusely</u>.

   The <u>well</u>-developed infant was <u>quite</u> talkative.

Verb Infinitive	Past Tense Form	Past Participle Form
become	became	become
begin	began	begun
break	broke	broken
bring	brought	brought
choose	chose	chosen
come	came	come
do	did	done
draw	drew	drawn
drink	drank	drunk
drive	drove	driven
eat	ate	eaten
find	found	found
forget	forgot	forgotten
get	got	gotten
give	gave	given
go	went	gone
hold	held	held
know	knew	known
lay	laid	laid
lead	led	led
leave	left	left
lie (to recline)	lay	lain
ring	rang	rung
rise	rose	risen
say	said	said
sew	sewed	sewn
see	saw	seen
sing	sang	sung
sit	sat	sat
speak	spoke	spoken
spring	sprang	sprung
stand	stood	stood
steal	stole	stolen
swim	swam	swum
take	took	taken
tear	tore	torn
write	wrote	written

Figure 9–6   Common irregular verbs

Articles

An **article** is a determiner that indicates a noun will follow. The three articles are the words *a, an,* and *the.* The articles *a* and *an* are often confused; use *a* for a noun beginning with a consonant or consonant sound and use *an* for a noun beginning with a vowel or vowel sound. Also, use *an* with a soft *h* sound, as in the words *historical* and *histologic.*

> *Examples:*   The physician is on call.
> A clamp is an important surgical instrument.
> A fine-needle biopsy can be a necessary part of making an
>   histologic assessment.

9–F Clauses and Phrases

Clauses

A **clause** is a group of related words containing a subject and a predicate that is not a complete sentence. Clauses are often set off from other parts of a sentence or other clauses by prepositions, conjunctions and clause introducers. A clause usually cannot stand on its own as a complete sentence because of its clause introducer.

> *Examples:*   The surgical intern who performed the operation was
>   undertrained.
> Although the risks were great, the procedure was necessary.
> The syllabus, which was part of the curriculum, was
>   lengthy.

A special note on clauses:

The words *that* and *which* are special clause introducers that are frequently confused in transcription. *That* always introduces **restrictive clauses**—clauses that are necessary to keep the meaning of the sentence intact. *Which* should be used to introduce only **nonrestrictive clauses** (clauses that are nonessential to preserve the meaning of the sentence, but provide additional information), although in a few cases *which* could also introduce a restrictive clause. Generally, however, use *that* to introduce restrictive clauses and *which* to introduce nonrestrictive clauses. If these words are found incorrectly interchanged in reports you transcribe, try to correct them.

> *Examples:*   The patient was a passenger in the automobile accident that
>   resulted in her paralysis.
>   (It is important to know that the automobile accident
>   resulted in her paralysis.)
> The patient injured her cervical spine in the accident, which
>   occurred two weeks ago.
>   (The fact that the accident occurred two weeks ago is
>   incidental; focus of the sentence is that the patient
>   injured her cervical spine in the accident.)

Phrases

A **phrase** is a group of related words lacking either a subject or a predicate. Although phrases are not complete sentences by themselves, they often stand alone, as would a sentence in medical transcription, especially when used under categories such as review of systems, physical examination, or laboratory data. In these cases, a phrase is often used to convey the meaning of a complete sentence as a component of a list.

Examples: According to the physician's assistant, the lab tests were not completed.

Tonsillectomy being indicated, the risks and complications were discussed.

She worked all day coding and abstracting reports.

Lungs: Without rales, wheezes or rhonchi. Genitalia: Normal male. Rectal: Deferred on this examination.

Some special notes on phrases:

Two special types of phrases are verbal and prepositional. A **verbal phrase** is comprised of a verb and all words related to it. A **prepositional phrase** is a phrase containing a preposition. Neither of these phrases should stand alone as a sentence except when used in a report under a category to describe its components or features, as in the last example.

Verbal phrase (that should not stand alone): Assessing patients' complaints

Sentence containing verbal phrase: Assessing patients' complaints is necessary for adequate evaluation.

Prepositional phrase (that should not stand alone): Toward the dorsal side.

Sentence containing prepositional phrase: The sutures were placed toward the dorsal side.

9–G Word Connectors: Conjunctions and Prepositions

Conjunctions

A **conjunction** joins one part of a sentence to another. Conjunctions link words, phrases and clauses. The words *and, but, or, nor, for, so* and *yet* are **coordinating conjunctions** that always connect two or more nouns, verbs, adjectives, adverbs, phrases or clauses.

Examples: The midwife or the nurse practitioner will assist the patient.

Strep and staph are two types of infectious processes.

The patient was prepped, but he was not intubated.

Prepositions

Prepositions also are connecting words. A preposition describes the relationship of something to something else. Some common prepositions follow:

about	above	across	after	against
along	among	around	as	at

before	behind	below	beneath	beside
between	beyond	by	despite	down
during	for	from	in	inside
into	like	near	next to	of
off	on	onto	out	out of
outside	over	past	round	since
through	throughout	to	toward	under
underneath	unlike	until	up	upon
with	within	without		

Some rules for prepositions:

1. Prepositions should come before their objects.
2. Try not to begin a sentence with a prepositional phrase.
3. Try not to end a sentence with a preposition.

9–H Special Grammar Notes

1. Use "were" with most statements expressing desire, or with statements beginning with "if."

   > *Examples:*   If I were a doctor, I would find a cure for many life-
   > threatening diseases.
   > I wish Dr. Higginbotham were my primary care physician.

2. Recognize the passive voice; in medical transcription, only change the passive voice to the active voice when the person who performs the action is known and is important to the sentence, or when the sentence is awkward in the passive voice.

   > Passive voice: The results of the test were thought to be nondiagnostic by the physician.
   >
   > Active voice: The physician thought the results of the test were nondiagnostic.

   > *Examples of when you should leave the passive voice as is:*
   > The operation was performed. (It is not important who performed the operation in this sentence.)
   > Under general anesthesia, the patient was prepped and draped in the normal sterile fashion. (It is not important who did the prepping and draping of the patient in this sentence.)
   > The octogenarian was seen by the visiting nurse when she went home. (The nurse is less important than the patient in this sentence.)

3. Be sure to always use the verb forms of *lie, lay, sit* and *set* correctly. *Lie* and *sit* are **intransitive verbs,** which cannot take objects. Intransitive verbs are used to show the action of persons or other living things. *Lay* and *set* are **transitive verbs** and almost always take objects. Transitive verbs are used to indicate that something is being done to an object.

   > *Examples:*   Pregnant patients are to lie down and take naps every afternoon.

You should have <u>laid</u> the reports on the radiologists' desks
for signatures.

The bird always <u>sits</u> on the ledge outside the patient's room.

Next time, please <u>try</u> to <u>set</u> the gurney down without such
force.

4. Ensure that subjects and verbs agree in number.

   a. When subjects are joined by the conjunction *and,* even if both are singular,
      use a plural verb.

      Examples: The scalpel <u>and</u> pursestring suture <u>rest</u> on the cart.

      Hemostats <u>and</u> electrocautery <u>are used</u> in operations.

   b. When subjects are joined by the conjunction *or,* the verb should agree with
      the closest subject.

      Examples: The pathologist <u>or the phlebotomists have called</u> in the
      report.

      Neither the physician <u>nor I like</u> the way the patient was
      treated.

   c. When modifying words come between subjects and verbs, the verb should
      agree with the main subject.

      Examples: The <u>physician.</u> as well as his nurses and assistants, <u>has</u>
      <u>volunteered</u> for the blood drive.

      The <u>profits earned</u> by one physician <u>were</u> donated to the
      orphanage.

5. Always try to make sentences and sentences within in a paragraph agree in
   tense and subject. For example, if the past tense is predominantly used
   throughout the paragraph, try not to use the present tense in a sentence in that
   same paragraph. Also make sure the subject is always clear and consistent.

   Examples: When this is dictated: "The exam <u>was</u> basically normal.
   The head, eyes, ears, nose and throat <u>were</u> negative, the
   throat <u>shows</u> no exudates."

   Type: "The exam <u>was</u> basically normal. The head, eyes,
   ears, nose and throat <u>were</u> negative; the throat
   <u>showed</u> no exudates."

   When this is dictated: "The patient was advised to see his
   physician, Dr. Smith, in 10 days, as <u>he</u> would be out of
   town next week."

   Type: "The patient was advised to see his physician,
   Dr. Smith, in 10 days, as <u>Dr. Smith</u> would be out of
   town next week."

Summary of Concepts

- Often, when dictating medical records, physicians and other dictators overlook
  basic parts of speech and incorrectly use sentence grammar; therefore, it is
  important that a medical transcriptionist become especially proficient at sentence grammar.

- It is especially important for transcriptionists to become familiar with classifications and cases of pronouns, because dictators often use them incorrectly when dictating.
- Indefinite pronouns always take singular pronouns.
- Indefinite pronouns usually take a singular verb, but the indefinite pronouns *all, any, none* and *some* may take a plural verb.
- It is important for a medical transcriptionist to become familiar with irregular verb forms, because dictators sometimes use the wrong irregular verb or verb form.
- If the words *that* and *which* are incorrectly interchanged in reports that are to be transcribed, the medical transcriptionist should try to correct them.
- A prepositional phrase or verb phrase should not stand alone as a sentence.
- Prepositions should come before their objects; try not to begin or end a sentence with a preposition.
- Use *were* with most statements expressing desire, or with statements beginning with *if*.
- The medical transcriptionist should be able to recognize the passive voice and change it to the active voice when necessary.
- The correct verb forms of *lie, lay, sit* and *set* should always be used.
- Always ensure that subjects and verbs agree in number.
- Always try to make sentences and sentences within in a paragraph agree in tense and subject; make sure the subject is always clear and consistent.

Chapter 10

Punctuation

Overview: Punctuation is the marking or dividing of words, groups of words or sentences with signs and symbols, such as periods, commas or semicolons, to mark the end of a thought. The correct use of punctuation is crucial for the medical transcriptionist, since most dictators of medical records do not bother to include punctuation, or when they do include it, it is oftentimes incorrect. Use this chapter as a guide for when and where to use punctuation marks.

Key Words

apostrophe	parentheses
asterisk	parenthesis mark
brackets	period
colon	question mark
comma	quotation marks
dash	semicolon
ellipsis	slash
exclamation point	virgule
hyphen	

10–A The Period

A **period** (.) is a point or dot used to mark the end of a sentence. In keyed reports, one sentence is separated from another after the period by two spaces. Use periods in the following cases:

1. to end sentences that are statements, mild commands or indirect questions
    Examples: The nurse was kind.
                      Follow the doctor's instructions.
                      The patient wondered why he was given the medication.

2. with many abbreviations
   Examples: M.D.
                     Ph.D.
                     p.m.
3. to separate dollars and cents, and to separate whole numbers and decimal fractions
   Examples: The cost of the seminar was $140.50.
                     Her hematocrit count was 42.5 on admission.
                     The specimen measured 1.5 cm × 4.5 mm.
4. after Roman numerals, Arabic numerals and alphabetical letters used to enumerate items in an outline or a list
   Examples: I. Laboratory Data
                         A. Blood work
                             1. Complete blood count
                             2. BUN
                             3. Creatinine
                             4. Chemistry panel
                             5. WBC with differential
                         B. Urinalysis
                         C. Toxicology screen
                     II. Physical Examination
                         A. Head and neck
                         B. Trunk
                         C. Extremities
5. after each initial in a person's name
   Examples: Dr. J. Paul Richardson
                     M. M. Malik, R.N.
                     Jonas A. Salk, M.D.
6. after an abbreviation that is part of a company's official legal name
   Examples: Siemens, Inc.
                     John Adams & Assoc.
                     Dewey, Cheatam & Howe, Ltd.

10-B The Question Mark

A **question mark** (?) is a hook-shaped mark with a dot directly underneath. It is used to indicate the conclusion of a sentence that is a direct question. Like the period, in keyed reports one sentence is separated from another after a question mark by two spaces. Use question marks in the following cases:

1. after direct questions
   Examples: Do you know what the diagnosis was?
                     "Will my condition ever improve?" asked the patient.
2. within parentheses to indicate doubt regarding a word or phrase
   Examples: The surgery was performed in 1979(?).
                     She had (?) diverticulitis.

3. after each of a series of items calling for individual answers

    Examples: Did you find the chart interesting? the assessment plausible? the diagnoses accurate?

    The physician questioned the patient about his previous psychiatric admissions. One time? Two times? Three times? More?

10-C The Exclamation Point

An **exclamation point** (!) is a rounded, tapered upside-down "I"-shaped mark used after an interjection, exclamation or other indication of a strong word or sentiment. Like the period and question mark, in keyed reports one sentence is separated from another after an exclamation point by two spaces. Use an exclamation point after emphatic statements, interjections or strong commands.

Examples: Whew! That scalpel almost nicked me!

When the physician saw the suture, he shouted, "What is this!"

Call security!

10-D The Comma

A **comma** (,) is a small, low-set, hook-shaped mark used to separate certain words in a sentence. One space follows a comma, separating two words. Use commas in the following cases:

1. before a coordinating conjunction linking main clauses that contain both a subject and predicate

    Examples: The surgeon performed the operation, and the physician performed the examination.

    The scalpel was new, but the rest of the instruments had been used before.

2. to set off most introductory elements, an element that modifies a word or words in the main clause that follows

    Examples: If he were a civilized person, the doctor would not be so difficult to work with.

    Frustrated, the transcriptionist left a blank.

3. to set off nonrestrictive elements, clauses and phrases, nonrestrictive meaning elements that provide additional information about the word or words to which it applies, but does not limit the word or words

    Examples: Transcriptionists, who turn dictation into written words, are skilled professionals.

    (However: Transcriptionists who work hard will get raises [no commas].)

    Good grammar, which is essential to proper medical record transcription, oftentimes is not properly taught in elementary schools.

4. to set off nonrestrictive appositives (an appositive is a noun or noun substitute that renames and may substitute for another noun immediately preceding it)

Examples: Electrocautery, a surgical cutting instrument that employs
both heat and electricity, is often an important part of an
operation.
All her daughters, Susan, Donna and Janice, signed the
consent for the operation.

5. to set off parenthetical expressions

Examples: The chairman of the board, according to the physician,
should have a vote.
Some nurses, for example, work in hospitals.

6. to set off *yes* and *no,* tag questions, words of direct address and mild interjections

Examples: Yes, the psychiatrist has a point.
Some physicians act superhuman, don't they?

7. to set off absolute phrases

Examples: Their work completed, the anatomy students went home.
Her stitches, the ends being frayed and rough, made her
uncomfortable.

8. to set off phrases expressing contrast

Examples: The medical report needs less opinion, more fact.
Hospitals are places for the sick, not the lonely.

9. between items in a series, between coordinate adjectives, and between more than one directly modifying adjective

Examples: Food, rest and fluids are the best remedy for a cold.
The clerical position requires typing, answering phones,
filing records and preparing documents.
The dirty, rusty, dented scalpel made the physician wince.
(In this sentence the adjectives *dirty, rusty* and *dented* each modify the
noun *scalpel* and each could stand alone with *scalpel.* The overall
meaning of the sentence would not change if any one of these adjectives
were removed.)

Exceptions:
There was bilateral mild red rhinitis and a thick yellow purulent
discharge.
(In this sentence the adjectives *bilateral, mild* and *red* each further modify
each other and do not directly modify the noun *rhinitis.* In other words,
if any of these adjectives were removed, the meaning of the sentence
would change. Therefore, no commas should be used.)

The right high-frequency sensorineural hearing loss was a result of
presbycusis.
(In this sentence the adjectives *right, high-frequency* and *sensorineural*
further modify each other and do not directly modify the noun *loss.* If
any of these adjectives were removed, the meaning of the sentence
would change. Again, no commas should be used.)

10. with dates, addresses, place names and long numbers

Examples: The operation was performed on May 2, 1979.
A kilometer equals approximately 3,280 feet.

11. with quotations
    Examples: The girl said, "My stomach hurts."
                   "I brought the papers," the patient stated.
12. to prevent misreading
    Examples: When she found out, she left the hospital for good.
                   Employees who can, usually give some money to charity.

10–E The Colon

A **colon** (:) is a pair of dots or points, one situated on top of the other, used to direct attention to something following it. In keyed reports, a colon is followed by two spaces before the next word is keyed. Use colons in the following cases:

1. to introduce an explanatory phrase, clause, sentence or group of sentences
   Examples: Family History: Noncontributory, as the patient was
                  adopted.
                  The reason for the decision is obvious: she failed to follow
                  directions.
2. to introduce a series of words, phrases or clauses
   Examples: Please bring the following to the AAMT meeting: a book, a
                  pen and a pencil.
                  There are three major laboratory blood work tests: the
                  complete blood count test, the arterial blood gas test, and
                  the superior mesentery artery test.
3. to introduce lengthy material that must be set off from the rest of a sentence in
   a manner other than quotation marks
   Example: The Nightingale Pledge begins like this: I solemnly pledge
                  myself before God and in the presence of this assembly
                  to pass my life in purity and to practice my profession
                  faithfully.
4. to separate hours from minutes in the expression of standard time in numbers
   Example: The operation will begin at 8:00 A.M.
5. to follow a salutation in business correspondence
   Example: Dear Dr. Smith:

10–F The Semicolon

A **semicolon** (;) is a mark containing a dot and a comma, with the comma situated under the dot, used to separate major portions of sentences. Only one space is used after a semicolon. Use semicolons in the following cases:

1. to separate main clauses not joined by a coordinating conjunction
   Examples: The boy was sick; he had a fever.
                  Some physicians speak clearly; others muffle their speech
                  and are hard to understand.
2. to separate main clauses related by a conjunctive adverb (consequently, hence,
   however, indeed, instead, nonetheless, otherwise, still, then, therefore and thus)

Examples: He was ill; therefore, he received treatment.

She is to return for follow-up in two weeks; however, if she has any complaints before that time she is to call the office.

3. to separate main clauses if they are long and complex, or if they contain commas, even when they are joined by a coordinating conjunction

Examples: He was cyanotic, pale and diaphoretic; and his wife brought him into the hospital.

The patient brought the following to the hospital: a gown; toiletries including a toothbrush and toothpaste, a comb and deodorant; and the surgery consent forms.

4. between an independent clause and a transitional expression such as "for example", "that is", "namely", "instead" or "for instance" when the expression precedes a list or another independent clause

Examples: A food challenge involves removing foods from the diet that are likely to contain allergens; for example, you should refrain from eating eggs for one week, milk for one week, grains for one week, etc.

The patient described several episodes of partial regurgitation; that is, he suffered from gastric reflux.

10–G The Apostrophe

An **apostrophe** (') is a high-set, comma-shaped mark used to indicate omission of characters or digits, the possessive case, and the plural forms of single characters, digits or figures. Use apostrophes in the following cases:

1. before or after an "s" ending to indicate the possessive case for nouns and indefinite pronouns

Examples: One must make one's own choices.

The twins' signs were consistent with their symptoms.

2. to indicate the omission of one or more letters, numbers or words in a standard contraction

Examples: It's time for the operation you're supposed to have.

The incision was made at the 3 o'clock position.

3. to form the plurals of letters, number and words named as words

Examples: Please do not forget to dot your i's and cross your t's when transcribing medical records.

The physician always confuses her a's and an's.

10–H Quotation Marks

Quotation marks (" ") are two sets of paired apostrophes used to indicate the beginning and end of a quotation. Sometimes a pair of single quotation marks (' ') is also used. Use quotation marks in the following cases:

1. to enclose direct quotations (use single quotation marks to enclose a quotation within a quotation)

[Note: Place commas and periods inside quotation marks, place colons and semicolons outside quotation marks, and place other punctuation inside quotation marks only if they belong in the quotation. Also, place commas and periods outside quotation marks when used with single letters or single words.]

> *Examples:*   "The insurance premium," the clerk explained, "has not been paid."
> "She told me 'my stomach hurts' after she swallowed the pill," the physician said.
> The patient complained of "cramping".

2. to enclose words or phrases that are slang or believed to be someone else's words

> *Examples:*   The patient said that she had taken several "uppers and downers" before coming to the emergency room.
> Joseph thought he was "king" of the psychiatric unit.
> After I began my exam, the patient stated that she had a "belly-ache".

3. around titles such as songs, short poems, articles in periodicals, short stories, essays, episodes of television and radio programs, and subdivisions of books

> *Examples:*   The patient often sang "London Bridge is Falling Down."
> Watch the episode "Diary of a Prostitute" on the *Oprah Winfrey Show* today.
> Shakespeare's "Hamlet" is a notable example of English literature.
> Please read Chapter 2, "Medical Transcription Transcribing Tools."

10–1 Other Punctuation Marks

The Dash   A **dash** (— or - -) is one long or two short flat marks situated together and used to separate certain parts of a sentence or thought. Use a dash:

to indicate an abrupt change in tone or thought
> *Example:*   The decision—not any easy one to make—was final.

to set off parts of some sentences
> *Example:*   Forceps, scalpels, sutures—these are some of the tools of surgery.

The Hyphen.   A **hyphen** (-) is a flat mark similar to a dash, also used to separate certain parts of a word, sentence or phrase. Use a hyphen:

to separate a word at the end of a line
> *Example:*   Although the patient's differential diagnosis included both osteoporosis and costochondritis, she had never previously been hospitalized.

between some prefix and root combinations
> *Example:*   He had a non-English accent.

in some compound words
> *Example:*   His mother-in-law lacked self-motivation.

to avoid ambiguity

    Example: She had a small-bowel exam. (versus: She had quite a small bowel.)

to indicate separation of the first and second parts of a hyphenated compound word group

    Example: She was given pre- and post-surgical instructions.

when it is necessary to write out compound numbers between 21 and 99

    Example: Thirty-two physicians were present at the symposium.

when writing out fractions, when they act as modifiers

    Example: A two-thirds majority of the pathologists voted "yea" at the meeting.

to replace the word *to* when used as a range between numerals

    Example: He is to return to the clinic in 10-14 days.

Further rules regarding hyphenation are discussed in Chapter 11.

Parentheses   **Parentheses** consist of two **parenthesis marks,** { (and) }, two opposite-facing curved lines used to indicate the beginning and end of one part of a sentence or phrase set off from another part. Use parentheses:

to enclose nonessential words, clauses or phrases that would not alter the meaning of a sentence. Use a single parenthesis to indicate numerical order.

    Examples: Motor vehicles (cars, for example) must yield to ambulances.

                      The patient is discharged on these medications: 1) estrogen, 2) hydrochlorothiazide, and 3) a Proventil inhaler.

to enclose symbols or figures that illustrate, clarify or confirm a word or word groups meaning

    Examples: Use an **asterisk** (*) to indicate that there is a footnote at the bottom of the page.

                      The reimbursement for the insured should have been at a rate of five percent (5%) instead of two percent (2%).

Brackets   **Brackets** consist of two marks ([and]), two opposite-facing curved lines, pointed in the middle, also used to indicate the beginning and end of one part of a sentence or phrase set off from another part. Use brackets within quotations to indicate editorial comments or changes, or with a word or group of words within a parenthetical phrase that would otherwise be set off with parentheses.

    Examples: "The patient [previously known to be uncooperative] was inebriated," he said.

                      (Please make corrections [if necessary] here.)

                      They died with there [sic] boots on.

Ellipses   An **ellipsis** (. . .), also indicated by the plural word *ellipses,* is a set of three or more spaced dots indicating omissions within quotations, to mark an unfinished sentence, or to separate text.

Examples: "I am nervous and cold . . . and confused," the patient stated.
A . . . . 10 points

The Slash   A **slash** (/), also called a **virgule,** is a diagonal mark used to separate two options or alternatives, or to represent the word *per* in abbreviations

Examples: This is a pass/fail course.
The dosage is 20 mg/kg.

Summary of Concepts

- The medical transcriptionist should become familiar with the following major punctuation marks and their uses: periods, question marks, exclamation points, commas, colons, semicolons, apostrophes and quotation marks.
- The medical transcriptionist should know when to use the following minor punctuation marks: dashes, hyphens, parentheses, asterisks, brackets, ellipses and slashes.

Chapter 11

Compound Words and Hyphenation

Overview: Why is it necessary for the medical transcriptionist to become familiar with compound and hyphenated words? Compound words present several challenges for the transcriptionist: Is the word an accepted compound word? Should the word parts be joined together or separated? Would it be better form to use hyphenation with the word or to avoid it? Some general rules for correctly forming compound and other commonly hyphenated words are discussed in this chapter.

Key Words

ambiguity	consolidated compound
attributive adjective	hyphenated compound
compound	hyphenation
compound adjective	open compound
compound noun	permanent compound
compound preposition	predicate adjective
compound verb	temporary compound
compound word	

11–A Compound Words and Hyphens

A **compound word,** or **compound,** is a word or word group consisting of two or more basic words or word parts, grouped together, to convey a specific idea. Sometimes the two or more combined words or word parts form one new word without punctuation, and sometimes a hyphen combines the words or word parts to form a new hyphenated word. Compound words can often be found in a dictionary.

As with other punctuation, the dictator usually does not mention in his or her dictation when and how a compound word group should be combined, so a medical transcriptionist must know exactly how to punctuate compounds. Not all dictators follow set rules; consult the dictator, when necessary, about his or her preferences regarding punctuating compounds.

There are several types of compounds. An explanation and examples of each type of compound, with pertinent rules when applicable, follow.

11–B Consolidated Compounds

A **consolidated compound** is a compound formed by joining one or more words or word parts without a hyphen.

Examples: a longstanding problem
mouthwash
a headache

Rules for consolidated compounds:

1. Words that have become common in usage are generally consolidated.
2. Consolidated compounds can often be found in dictionaries.

11–C Hyphenated Compounds

A **hyphenated compound** is a compound formed by joining one or more words or word parts with a hyphen.

Examples: an oral-antral fistula
the water-bottle
year-end reconciliation

Rules for hyphenated compounds:

1. If unsure about using a consolidated or hyphenated compound and the compound cannot be located in a dictionary, use hyphenation as a fail-safe method of forming the compound.
2. Use a hyphen with a compound to avoid confusion, to avoid **ambiguity** (conveying an unclear or indistinct meaning), or to avoid making an awkward combination of letters, especially with the following prefixes: *ante-, anti-, bi-, co-, contra-, counter-, de-, inter-, intra-, macro-, micro-, mid-, non-, out-, over-, post-, pre-, pro-, pseudo-, re-, semi-, sub-, super-, trans-, tri-, ultra-, un-.*

Examples: re-creation (again created) vs. recreation (leisure activity)
[hyphenation in the first case avoids confusion]
re-enactment vs. reenactment
[hyphenation in the first case avoids the placement of two identical vowels together, which would be awkward]
childlike vs. pill-like
[lack of hyphenation would make "pill-like" have three consonants together, which would be an awkward combination of letters]
pre-enteric vs. preenteric
[lack of hyphenation would make the word awkward and difficult to pronounce]

3. Use a hyphen to combine compounds when the second word part begins with a capital letter:
   Examples: anti-American
   non-Catholic
   pre-Civil War
4. Use hyphenated compounds when numerical expressions are used as parts of compound words.
   Examples: one-year history
   a 3-month-old girl
5. Use a hyphenated compound when a word is a compound noun but is used as an implied compound adjective.
   Examples: The 6-year-old came into the office. [a missing noun such as "child" is implied]
   The three-inch was preferred to the two-inch. [a missing noun such as "stitch" is implied]
6. Use hyphenation to clarify meaning or make pronunciation easier.
   Examples: It was a small bowel loop causing the abnormality in the lower intestine. [refers to a bowel loop that is little in size]
   vs.
   The abnormality seen was a small-bowel loop. [refers to the small bowel of the intestine]
7. Use hyphenation when awkward or ambiguous doubled letters would result from a typically consolidated compound, or to make pronunciation of a compound easier.
   Examples: post-traumatic [instead of posttraumatic]
   re-x-ray [instead of rex-ray]
8. Use hyphenation with compounds that would normally be consolidated but include abbreviations.
   Examples: pre-CABG instructions
   non-PID disorder

11–D Open compounds

An **open compound** is a compound formed when two words or word parts are associated without being joined.
   Examples: chopping block
   chest cold
   heart attack

Rules for open compounds:

1. If a compound would cause too much attention to be directed to a word if hyphenated or consolidated, or if it would be confusing or distracting, use the open compound form.
   Example: He complained of stomach acid. [causes no confusion or distraction]
   not
   He complained of stomach-acid.

> *or*
>> He complained of stomachacid.
>>> [causes confusion and distraction]

2. Compound nouns formed from a present or past participle verb form and a noun should be open.

> *Examples:*   operating room
> jellied gauze

11–E Permanent Compounds

A **permanent compound** is a joined word that is so common in usage that it has become an established or a permanent part of the English language and is spelled as one word.

> *Examples:*   notwithstanding
> Nosebleeds and eardrops are sometimes related.
> nevertheless

Rules for permanent compounds:

1. Permanent compounds can often be found in dictionaries.
2. Permanent compounds usually are not hyphenated.

11–F Temporary Compounds

A **temporary compound** is the opposite of a permanent compound. It is a joined word that is coined or invented by an author or dictator to serve a specific, usually temporary, purpose. However, a dictator may also use the word frequently in dictation.

> *Examples:*   her ironing-board-stiff stomach
> a wait-and-monitor protocol
> a spur-of-the-moment decision

Rules for temporary compounds:

1. Temporary compounds usually are not found in a dictionary.
2. Temporary compounds usually are joined with a hyphen.
3. Sometimes the meaning of a temporary compound is apparent only to the dictator.
4. Some temporary compounds are familiar and have been in common usage for some time; however, these temporary compounds are still considered informal and have not yet been categorized in a dictionary, thus they are still hyphenated when written.

11–G Compound Nouns

A **compound noun** is a compound consisting of words or word parts. A compound noun functions as a noun in a sentence. It can be consolidated, hyphenated or open.

Examples: cottonball
                     health-mobile
                     time off

Rules for compound nouns:

1. As temporary compound nouns become permanent, they also become consolidated.
    Examples: spread sheet (temporary) vs. spreadsheet (permanent)
                      breast feed (temporary) vs. breastfeed (permanent)
2. Compound nouns that are formed with the suffixes *-man, -men, -woman, -women, -person* or *-people* usually are consolidated instead of hyphenated.
    Examples: saleswoman
                      spokesperson

11–H Compound Adjectives

A **compound adjective** is a compound consisting of words or word parts that functions as an adjective or a noun modifier in a sentence.
    Examples: a well-developed infant
                      a medical school graduate
                      The medication was fast acting.

Rules for compound adjectives:

1. When a compound adjective is an **attributive adjective,** or precedes the noun it modifies, use a hyphen to connect it (unless the first word is an adverb that ends in *ly*):
    Examples: She was a well-developed, well-nourished, under-educated
                         girl of 18.
                      She had a right high-frequency nerve loss.
                          but
                      It was a slowly draining abscess. [The first word of the
                         compound adjective is an adverb ending in -ly.]
2. When a compound adjective is a **predicate adjective,** or follows the noun it modifies along with the verb or predicate, do not use a hyphen.
    Examples: The baby appeared well developed.
                      Her fever became low grade.
3. Compound adjectives containing the suffix *-free* are hyphenated, whether preceding or following the noun it modifies.
    Examples: He had been symptom-free for six weeks.
                      Her ears were fluid-free.
4. Many temporary compound adjectives are formed when a three or more word phrase is hyphenated and positioned before a noun.
    Examples: She displayed a never-before-seen aggressiveness.
                      The soon-to-be-discharged patient picked up his
                         prescriptions.

11–I Compound Prepositions

A **compound preposition** is a compound group of words containing many prepositions. Compound prepositions usually are open. Clauses containing compound prepositions should be set off from the rest of a sentence with a comma.

Examples: In addition to the above, the patient was given diet modifications.

Beneath the line of type in the margins of the page, all the diagnoses were handwritten.

11–J Additional Rules for Compound Words

1. Compound words using the prefixes *self-* or *all-* or the suffixes *-elect* and *-free* should always be hyphenated.

   Examples: self-control   all-encompassing
                 self-image   all-inclusive
                 president-elect   member-elect
                 duty-free   complaint-free

2. Special rules apply when the words *follow-up, workup* and *checkup* are used as compounds.

   a. When the word is a compound used as a verb, or a **compound verb,** do not hyphenate.

      Examples: He is to follow up next week.
                    She had checked up the infant twice in a month.
                    All his symptoms were worked up.

   b. When the word is a compound adjective or noun, hyphenate or consolidate it.

      Examples: The patient is to be seen in follow-up next week.
                    The child was in for her yearly checkup.
                    The thorough workup included x-rays and a CT scan.

11–K General Rules for Hyphenation

Questions regarding **hyphenation,** or the placement of a hyphen to separate or combine words, often arise in the transcription process. Because the rules for hyphenating compounds and other words can be confusing, it is important for the medical transcriptionist to be able to identify a word that should be hyphenated and correctly use hyphenation.

Some general rules for hyphenation follow:

1. Use hyphenation for written fractions or compound numbers.

   Examples: An incision was made at the junction of the anterior one-third of the cord with the posterior two-thirds.

   She is to reduce the dosage by one-half. [or, She is to reduce the dosage by a half.]

2. Use hyphenation when spelling out the numbers twenty-one to ninety-nine.

   Examples: Twenty-one sagittal slices of the skull were made on CT scan.

   Seventy-nine percent of patients with this condition improve in a year or less.

3. Use hyphenation with suture sizes including 0s.

   Examples: The wound was closed with 3-0 Prolene.

   She used running 2-0 absorbable sutures for the subcutaneous tissue.

4. Use hyphenation when expressing ranges in numbers that are in numeral form. When the numbers in the ranges are spelled out, however, use the word *to* instead of a hyphen.

   Examples: The patient was to have the wound rechecked every 7-10 days.

   There were 24,000-48,000 WBCs seen on microscopic exam.

   The operation's cost was in the ballpark of $1,500-$2,500.

   but

   She has had the symptoms for two to three days.

5. Use hyphenation when forming attributive compound adjectives including numbers or when numbers are implied.

   Examples: She had a 20-db hearing deficit.

   A 15-cm incision was made into the peritoneum.

   There was a several-year history of diabetic retinopathy.

Summary of Concepts

- A compound is a word or word group consisting of two or more basic words or word parts, grouped together, conveying a specific idea.
- Sometimes the two or more combined words or word parts form one new word without punctuation, and sometimes a hyphen combines the words or word parts to form a new hyphenated word.
- Types of compound words include permanent and temporary compounds; consolidated, hyphenated and solid compounds; compound nouns, compound verbs, compound prepositions and compound adjectives. Compound adjectives can be either attributive or predicative.
- Hyphenation can be used to avoid awkward word or letter combinations, to avoid ambiguity, and with compounds containing numbers or numerical expressions.

Chapter 12

Contractions and Shortened Word Forms

Overview: With informal spoken or written expressions of thought, it is acceptable to use contractions. However, try to avoid them in medical transcription. Also, shortened word forms are often used as time-saving measures, but since they can sometimes lead to confusion on the part of the reader if transcribed incorrectly or inappropriately, a medical transcriptionist needs to be familiar with how and when to use contractions and shortened word forms.

Key Words

acceptable brief forms

apostrophized contractions

brief form

contractions

shortened word

shortened word forms

unacceptable brief forms

unapostrophized contractions

verb phrase contractions

12–A Contractions

What are contractions? **Contractions** are condensed forms of expressions. An apostrophe usually replaces the missing letters. Although in medical transcription contractions generally should not be used, it is helpful to know how contractions are formed and the rules for using them in transcription.

Some contractions are formed, or constructed, with an apostrophe, called **apostrophized contractions,** and other contractions are formed without them, called **unapostrophized contractions.** Following are examples of each.

1. **Apostrophized contractions:**
    Examples:
    it is → it's　　　　　　　　　were not → weren't
    they are → they're　　　　　　cannot → can't
    you are → you're　　　　　　　1988 → '88

who is → who's

does not → doesn't

of the clock → o'clock

madam → ma'am

2. **Unapostrophized contractions:**

Examples:

all + together → altogether

all + ready → already

all + though → although

through → thru

until → till

12–B Rules for Contractions

Following are some general rules for contractions used in medical transcription.

1. Try to avoid contractions in medical transcription. If the client you are transcribing for permits it, contractions may be used in informal records transcription such as office chart notes. However, when a physician dictates a contraction in formal correspondence, such as a letter, use the words that form the contraction instead of the contraction.

2. Be careful not to confuse contractions with plurals and possessives. In a contraction, there are missing letters when two or more words are combined. In a plural case, no letters are missing, but an "s" or an "'s" is added to make a single word or group of words plural. In a possessive case, no letters are missing, but an "'s" or simply an apostrophe is added to make a single word or group of words express ownership or possession. Also, do not confuse the personal pronouns "its", "their", "your" and "whose" with the contractions "it's", "they're", "you're" and "who's."

3. **Verb phrase contractions** (don't, weren't, isn't, aren't, etc.) are common in informal writing, but try not to use them in medical transcription; write out "do not", "were not", "is not", "are not" and so on, whenever possible.

Following are some specific rules pertaining to using apostrophes for contractions.

1. Sometimes there is confusion about whether or not to use a contraction when combining "all +" word combinations. If "all" means "each and every one," it should not become part of a contraction and should remain a single word.

Examples: We were all together.

vs.

We were not altogether sure of our reasoning.

[In the first sentence, "all together" means all of us were gathered in one place; in the second sentence, "altogether" means entirely or totally.]

We are all ready for the photo.

vs.

We had already discussed the matter.

[In the first sentence, "all ready" means all prepared or thoroughly prepared; in the second sentence, "already" means prior to the current time or before now.]

2. There is no contraction for the words "all right" and "a lot." These word groups should always be written as two words.

12–C Shortened Word Forms

Lengthy or complex medical terms are often shortened when used in spoken or written medical dialect. Sometimes these words are shortened in the form of a contraction, with or without an apostrophe, or in the form of an abbreviation, with one or more periods (which will be fully explained in the following chapter). Other times these words are shortened simply by removing a few key letters, letters that often are not critical to retain the meaning of the word, and condensing the remaining letters into a shorter word. The resulting **shortened word,** or shortened form of the word, is also called a **brief form.** A shortened word can be called a "slang" term as well.

12–D Acceptable and Unacceptable Shortened Word Forms

Some **shortened word forms** are acceptable in medical transcription, while others are not. Following are examples of both types of shortened word forms.

1. **Acceptable brief forms.** Because some shortened words are commonplace and accepted throughout the English medical language as acceptable shortened word forms, and usually do not run the risk of being confused with other similar words or word forms, certain words are acceptable for use as brief forms. The following brief word forms are usually acceptable, except if dictated in full form or if the physician's or hospital's style necessitates that the word form be written out in full form.

examination → exam	Papanicolaou smear → Pap smear
laboratory → lab	postoperative → postop
prepared → prepped	sedimentation rate → sed rate
prepare/preparation → prep	influenza → flu
preoperative → preop	prothrombin time → pro time
streptococcus → strep	staphylococcus → staph

2. **Unacceptable brief forms.** Because some shortened words could be confused by the reader for other words, or lose their clarity when shortened, they should not be used in their shortened word or brief form in medical transcription. Do not use brief forms for the following words; always spell out the complete word.

subcutaneous/subcuticular (subcu)	palpable or palpation (palp)
laparotomy/laparoscopy (lap)	capsules/capital letters (caps)
electrolytes (lytes)	prescription (script)
calculated (calc)	tablets (tabs)

differential (diff)   chemical (chem)
appendectomy (appy)   medications/medicines (meds)
dexamethasone (dex)   saturation (sat)
bilirubin (bili)   audiogram/audiology (audio)

The following two brief forms are becoming more acceptable in usage. Check with the facility or dictator for which you are transcribing to see whether or not it would be appropriate to use them.

temperature (temp)   vital signs (vitals)

Summary of Concepts

- Understand what contractions are and when and how to use them in medical transcription.
- Become familiar with apostrophized and unapostrophized contractions.
- Know what shortened word and brief word forms are.
- Recognize acceptable and unacceptable brief or shortened word forms.

Chapter 13

Abbreviations

Overview: Using abbreviations can be an asset or a liability to the medical transcriptionist. Sometimes abbreviations are used as time-savers by the dictator, are well known, and are acceptable for use in medical transcription. Other times they are not well known, are unclear or ambiguous, or are simply not appropriate for use in a specific medical transcription setting. An explanation of how, when, and which abbreviations should or should not be used in the transcription of medical dictation follows.

Key Words

abbreviations

courtesy titles

geographic names

Latin abbreviations

lowercase abbreviations

mixed-case abbreviation

professional titles

social titles

units of measure

uppercase abbreviations

13–A What Are Abbreviations?

Abbreviations, like shortened and brief word forms, are condensed versions of words. Some abbreviations use periods, some use capital letters standing alone, and some use both periods and small letters. Although abbreviations should never be used simply to avoid transcribing lengthy words or material, they are commonly used in medical transcription. Therefore, thoroughly familiarize yourself with the proper forms of abbreviations and some common forms they can take. Abbreviations and the words they stand for often can be found in medical or standard English dictionaries.

In addition to learning the guidelines on abbreviations in medical reports, be aware that every accredited hospital is required by the major hospital accrediting agency, the Joint Commission on Accreditation (JCAH), to keep on file a list of acceptable abbreviations for that institution. The only abbreviations appearing in that facility's medical records and reports should be those which are on the Approved Abbreviations List. Check with the medical facility for whom you are working to see if it has an Approved Abbreviations List, and be sure to use only those abbreviations on the list and spell out the words otherwise.

13–B General Rules for Abbreviations

1. **Acceptable uses of abbreviations.** It is generally acceptable to use abbreviations in the following circumstances:

   with most quantity measurements
   Examples:
   > 24 cm long
   > 1 g specimen
   > 10 lb. infant

   with most laboratory data [See Appendix F for further explanation.]
   Examples:
   > CBC, not Complete Blood Count
   > SMAC, not Superior Mesenteric Artery Count
   > ESR, not Estimated Sedimentation Rate

   with Latin abbreviations (also, always use commas before, with a space, and after these abbreviations)
   Examples:
   > e.g.
   > etc.
   > i.e., H. Brown, Smith, B., et al.

   with percentages, only when the numeral directly precedes the unit of measure or when the numeral and percentage together reflect a result or score of diagnostic laboratory data
   Examples:
   > 15%
   >   but, 15 mg percent
   > a 10% FEV/FVC ratio
   >   but, "There was a 10 percent increase in the lung capacity volume."
   > "His discrimination score in the left ear was 20%."
   >   but, "His hearing loss had dropped 20 percent."

   with chemical symbols when contained in laboratory data, or when they include units of measure
   Examples:
   > Lab data: His K was 2.0 and his Na was 123.
   > Test results showed 60 mm Hg.
   > "There was no NaCl found on urinalysis."

when expressing abbreviated unit measurements including "per" with a slash

Examples:
15 mm/dl
20 mg/day
30 kg/year of age

2. **Unacceptable uses of abbreviations.** It is generally unacceptable to use abbreviations in the following circumstances:

in diagnoses, impressions, assessments or in the names of operative procedures

Examples:
FINAL DIAGNOSIS: Hemophilus influenza
(not "H. influenza," if dictated this way)
NAME OF OPERATION: Thoracic outlet cutdown, three millimeters in
length
(not "3 mm")
IMPRESSION: Negative Papanicolaou smear
(not "Pap smear," if dictated)

at the beginning of a sentence, except with personal name and courtesy titles

Examples:
The pH testing was within normal limits.
(not "pH testing was within normal limits.")
Four cubic centimeters of the fluid were extracted
(not "4 cc of the fluid were extracted.")
A CT scan was performed.
or
Computerized tomography scan was performed.
(not "CT scan was performed.")

in measurements, when the quantity is unknown

Examples:
several milligrams
a few centimeters
no grams of fat
(but "0 g. fat" is acceptable)

if the abbreviation is not dictated

Examples:
If "total abdominal hysterectomy/bilateral salpingo-oophorectomy" is
dictated, do not abbreviate the word "TAH-BSO."
If "three times a day" is dictated, do not abbreviate "t.i.d."
If "red blood cells" is dictated, do not abbreviate "RBCs."

with days of the week or names of months

Examples:
March 1, 1996
(not Mar. 1, 1996)
Friday the 3rd
(not Fri. the 3rd)

<u>September through December</u>
(not Sept.–Dec.)

on the first reference of most companies' names, organizations' names, and on the first reference to genus name

Examples:

On first reference to "TENS unit" type "<u>transcutaneous electrical nerve stimulation unit</u>"; thereafter, abbreviate.

On first reference to "AIDS" type "<u>acquired immunodeficiency syndrome</u>"; thereafter abbreviate.

On first reference to "AT&T" type "<u>American Telegraph and Telephone</u>"; thereafter, abbreviate.

with certain laboratory data [See Appendix F for further information.]

Examples:

<u>eosinophils</u> (not "eos")
<u>reticulocytes</u> (not "retics")
<u>hemoglobin and hematocrit</u> (not H&H)

with most chemical symbols, such as K for potassium, Pb for lead, C for carbon, and so on, in the body of the transcription, other than in laboratory data (however, O_2 and all forms and combinations including oxygen are acceptable to abbreviate everywhere but in a diagnosis)

Examples:

The patient's <u>lead</u> levels were high on the day of admission.
(not "The patient's Pb levels were high . . .")
He had low serum <u>potassium</u> before electrolytes administration.
(not "IIe had low serum K before electrolytes . . .")
The patient responded well to nasal $\underline{O_2}$. (acceptable)

13–C Uppercase Abbreviations

1. Usually **uppercase,** or capitalized, **abbreviations** do not take periods in their forms. When they are made plural, a simple lowercase "s" should be added, not an apostrophe + "s" ('s)

    Examples: <u>CT</u> scan
    The <u>CBC</u> showed 15,000 <u>WBCs</u>.
    <u>URIs</u>

2. Use uppercase abbreviations with numbers:

    Examples: <u>2PD</u>—two-point discrimination
    <u>5FU</u>—5-fluorouracil
    <u>3D</u>—three-dimensional

13–D Lowercase Abbreviations

1. Usually **lowercase,** or small, not capitalized, **abbreviations** take periods in their forms, except in units of measurement. When the latter are made plural, periods should be deleted and an apostrophe + "s" should be added ('s).

    Examples: p.r.n.

no erythema o.d. or o.l.
She was given the medication in the am's instead of the pm's.

2. **Latin abbreviations,** abbreviations incorporating Latin terms, usually are lower-case and take periods. These abbreviations should be preceded and followed by commas when used in writing. Some common Latin abbreviations follow:

cf.	compare
e.g.	for example
etc.	and so forth; and other things
et seq.	and the following
et al.	and others (often used in source citations)
i.e.	that is; in other words
ibid.	in the same place (often used to indicate the same book or page in source citations)
id.	the same (often used to indicate repetition of an author's name or title in source citations)

13–E Mixed Case Abbreviations

Usually **mixed case abbreviations,** abbreviations that use a combination of uppercase and lowercase letters, do not take periods in their forms. Many chemical symbols also use mixed-case abbreviations (see Figure 13–1). When mixed-case abbreviations are made plural, add a simple lowercase "s" if the abbreviation ends in an uppercase letter, or add an apostrophe + "s" ('s) if the abbreviation ends in a lowercase letter.

Examples: Pb poisoning
The pHs were high.
Their Hx's were unremarkable.

13–F Units of Measure

Units of measure are the words or abbreviations following numerals describing weight, height, depth, length, or other ways to determine the specifics of something that can be measured. Generally, metric unit abbreviations use lower-case or mixed case without periods. English (avoirdupois) measurement units usually use lowercase abbreviations with periods.

Metric Abbreviation	Long Metric Unit of Measure
ng, nl, nm	nanogram, nanoliter, nanometer
mcg, mcl, mcm	microgram, microliter, micrometer
mg, ml, mm	milligram, milliliter, millimeter
cg, cl, cm	centigram, centiliter, centimeter
dg, dl, dm	decigram, deciliter, decimeter

Symbol	Chemical Name	Symbol	Chemical Name
Ag	silver	K	potassium
Al	aluminum	Kr	krypton
Am	americium	Li	lithium
Ar	argon	Mo	molybdenum
As	arsenic	N	nitrogen
Au	gold	Na	sodium
Ba	barium	Ne	neon
Be	beryllium	Ni	nickel
Bi	bismuth	O	oxygen
B	boron	P	phosphorus
Br	bromine	Pb	lead
C	carbon	Pt	platinum
Ca	calcium	Pu	plutonium
Cd	cadmium	Ra	radium
Ce	cerium	Rh	rhodium
Cl	chlorine	Rn	radon
Co	cobalt	S	sulfur
Cr	chromium	Sb	antimony
Cs	cesium	Se	selenium
Cu	copper	Si	silicon
Er	erbium	Sn	tin
F	fluorine	Tc	technetium
Fe	iron	Te	tellurium
Fr	francium	Ti	titanium
Ga	gallium	Tl	thallium
Gd	gadolinium	U	uranium
H	hydrogen	W	tungsten
He	helium	Xe	xenon
Hg	mercury	Y	yttrium
I	iodine	Yb	ytterbium
Ir	iridium	Zn	zinc
Mg	magnesium	Zr	zirconium
Mn	manganese		

Figure 13–1 Common chemical symbols

Metric Abbreviation	Long Metric Unit of Measure
g, l, m	gram, liter, meter
Dg, Dl, Dm	dekagram, dekaliter, dekameter
hg, hl, hm	hectogram, hectoliter, hectometer
kg, kl, km	kilogram, kiloliter, kilometer

English Abbreviation	Long English Unit of Measure
gr.	grain
oz.	ounce
lb.	pound
pt.	pint
qt.	quart
gal.	gallon
tsp.	teaspoon
tbsp.	tablespoon
in.	inch
ft.	foot
yd.	yard
mi.	mile
sec.	second
min.	minute
hr.	hour

13–G Abbreviations with Temperatures

When using abbreviations with temperatures, it is appropriate to use only the numeral to indicate degrees, if dictated. However, if either the term "degrees" or the words "Fahrenheit" or "Celsius" are used, both the word "degrees" and the type, either Fahrenheit or Celsius, must be written. Thus, a temperature of 100 in a febrile patient would be written as either "temperature was 100" or "temperature was 100 degrees Fahrenheit," but not "temperature was 100 degrees" or "temperature was 100 Fahrenheit."

13–H Abbreviations with Geographic Names

Rules for using abbreviations with **geographic names,** or names that describe places follow. In correspondence (letters), use abbreviations for direction (S., N., E., W., S.W., N.E., etc.), street (Ave., Dr., St., Cir., Blvd., etc.), state (use the postal abbreviations, such as CA [not Calif.], CO, TX, IA, ME, WA, etc.), and country (U.S.A., P.R.C., R.O.C.) if there is an acceptable abbreviation for the country. Commas precede and follow all cities with states (e.g., She has lived in Denver, Colorado, for three years). In formal reports, do not use geographic abbreviations.

13–I Abbreviations with Dates

Write out the days of the week and dates (Monday, January 19, 1999, instead of Mon., Jan. 19, '99 or Mon., 1/19/99). Commas precede and follow all dates. Use dashes instead of slashes with dates (1-19-99), unless it is the preferred style of the physician or hospital to do otherwise. Do not use ordinals (numbers used to show sequence in a series, such as 12*th*), except when they precede the month or stand alone (e.g., the 12th of March, or the 12th, but not March 12th).

13–J Abbreviations with Titles and Degrees

1. Always abbreviate **social titles** (**courtesy titles** such as Mr., Ms. or Mrs.) when they are used with names. Also, drop the courtesy title if a **professional title** (a title such as Dr.) is concurrently used.

    Examples: Mrs. Indira Khan, or Indira Khan, R.N.
    Ms. Lin Nguyen or Dr. Lin Nguyen, or Lin Nguyen, Ph.D.
    Mr. Richard Chang, or Richard Chang, M.A.
    Dr. Felix Delgado, or Felix Delgado, Ph.D.

2. Never concurrently use a social title before a name and a professional title afterward.

    Examples: Joe Littlebear, M.D. or Dr. Joe Littlebear, not Dr. Joe
    Littlebear, M.D.
    Luci Kamchatka P.A.-C or Ms. Luci Kamchatka, not
    Ms. Luci Kamchatka, P.A.-C

3. Use periods and no space when using a professional title.

    Examples: Kim Miyaki, M.D.
    Sue Szczescu, R.N.
    Hanna Johansen, R.M.T.
    Tasha Mutombe, B.A., M.A., Ph.D., M.D. (Always use the
    degree with the least educational requirements first.)

4. Abbreviate the following social titles when used before a name: Dr. (doctor), Gov. (governor), Lt. Gov. (lieutenant governor), Mr. (mister), Mrs. (mistress), Rep. (representative), Sen. (senator), Lt. (lieutenant), Col. (colonel), the Rev. (the Reverend), and so on.

13–K Abbreviations with Names, Sign-off Initials and Letter Notations

Use the following as a guide:
J. F. Kennedy, not J.F. Kennedy or JF Kennedy
RH/jmtsl, RH:jmtsl or jmtsl, not rh:JMTSl or rh:jmtsl
pc: (photocopy to) or cc: (carbon copy to), not PC or CC
Encl., enc. or Enclosures, not Enc.

Summary of Concepts

- Understand the cases in which abbreviations are acceptable for use in medical transcription.
- Understand the cases in which abbreviations are unacceptable for use in medical transcription.
- Know the rules and formats for uppercase, lowercase and mixed-case abbreviations.
- Become familiar with the common Latin abbreviations.
- Learn how to abbreviate units of measure.
- Recognize the rules for abbreviating with temperatures, geographic names, dates, and titles and degrees.
- Never abbreviate simply for expediency's sake.

Chapter 14

Capitalization

Overview: Knowing when and when not to capitalize a word or letters in a word can present a challenge for the medical transcriptionist. Should, for instance, a particular abbreviation be capitalized? Should a word following a colon be capitalized? The answers to questions such as these are not always clear. Therefore, it is essential that the medical transcriptionist understand the rules for capitalization.

Key Words

brand names

capitalize

eponym

genus

trade names

14–A General Rules for Letter Capitalization in Medical Transcription

1. **Capitalize,** or make uppercase, the first letter of the first word of every complete sentence.

    Examples: Two percent Xylocaine with epinephrine was used in the appendectomy.

    Examination of cranial nerves II through XII was not remarkable.

    Fifty-five out of one hundred patients do not develop the symptoms.

2. Capitalize the first letter of proper nouns, proper adjectives and other proper words. Also, capitalize the first letter of major words of a title.

    Examples: The patient, John Smith, lived in Los Angeles, California.

    Madame Curie was a French scientist.

Her Babinski's reflexes were normal.

"A Symptomatic Approach to Treatment of Vertigo in Patients with Meniere's Disease" was written by Jean Claude Basien, M.D.

3. Capitalize the first letter of the first word of a direct quotation involving a complete sentence, and capitalize the first letter of the first word in the first portion only of a quotation that is separated mid-sentence.

> *Examples:* She dictated, "The medication is to be taken p.r.n."
>
> "There are more patients in the waiting room," the clerk stated.
>
> "Because of fee capitation," the chairperson said, "we will no doubt suffer major financial cutbacks."

4. Capitalize the first word of a complete parenthetical sentence that stands alone (however, do not capitalize sentence fragments contained within a sentence).

> *Examples:* The plans are being finalized. (Carolyn should have a copy by Thursday.)
>
> Her physician was one of many at the conference (although he did not speak).

5. Capitalize the first word of salutations and complimentary closes of letters of correspondence. (Capitalize the first letter of each word with the salutation "To Whom It May Concern" and salutations referring to collective groups.)

> *Examples:* Dear Sirs:
>
> To Whom It May Concern:
>
> Ladies and Gentlemen:
>
> Sincerely,
>
> Best regards,

6. Capitalize only the first letters of words following periods when listing components of body systems in the Review of Systems or the Physical Examination. (Note: It is not necessary to use complete sentences in the Review of Systems and the Physical Examination.)

> *Examples:* Eyes: Clear. Pupils equal, round and reactive to light and accommodation; fundi normal; conjunctivae normal.
>
> Chest: Clear. No rhonchi, rales or rubs. There are no abnormal lung sounds.
>
> Heart: Normal sinus rhythm.

7. Place a capitalized article, pronoun or title before words that usually are not capitalized. Also, always insert an article before the word "patient" whenever it is dictated alone in a sentence.

> *Examples:* Mr. vanHuesen arrived well before his appointment time.
>
> The pH was 7.6; however, the specific gravity was 1.001.
>
> The patient was seen in his office.

8. Capitalize "I" when used as a pronoun and "O" when used as an interjection.

> *Examples:* The patient stated he was sick; however, I had my doubts.
>
> The song, "O Holy Night," rekindled old memories for the patient.

9. Capitalize the first letter of formal names of races, nationalities and languages, but do not capitalize informal descriptions of race by color.

Examples: The patient was a Caucasian female who spoke German
fluently.

He was a soft-spoken, black male, who was in no acute
distress.

She was a well-developed, well-nourished, Oriental woman.

10. Capitalize the first letter of a word following a colon only when the word stands alone or when the word begins a complete sentence. When a clause or phrase follows a colon that further explains text before the colon, it is not necessary to capitalize the first word of the clause or phrase.

Examples: Genitourinary examination: Normal.

Family History: Noncontributory.

Past History: The patient had the usual childhood illnesses.
He had a tonsillectomy at age 8 and an adenoidectomy at
age 9.

The patient had the following complaints: nausea,
diaphoresis and two-pillow orthopnea.

11. Capitalize the first letter of formal names of diseases, **eponym** (diseases named after a person) and the **genus** (a classification between family and species), group or family name of disease processes, but do not capitalize informal disease processes.

Examples: DISCHARGE DIAGNOSES:
1. Chronic Hemophilus influenzae
2. Past history of Crohn's disease
3. Status post myocardial infarction
4. Chronic diabetes mellitus
5. End-stage leukemia

12. Capitalize the first letter of the first word of a genus/species name when followed by a family name (see Figure 14–1). If the genus/species name is not followed by a family name, it may be lowercase. Also, always make the family name lowercase.

Examples: Aerobacter aerogenes
Clostridium tetani
The diagnosis was candida.

13. Roman numerals usually are capitalized when used in text. Use lowercase Roman numerals only as subnumerals with data recording or when outlining a report, research paper, and so on.

Examples: Cranial nerves II through XII were intact. She was gravida I
para I AB 0.

   I. Common symptoms
     A. Subjective
       1. Headache
       2. Stomachache
       3. Nausea
       4. Painful musculoskeletal area
         a. limb
           i. arm
           ii. leg

Genus/Species Name	Genus with Family Name (example)
actinomyces	Actinomyces muris
amoeba	Amoeba urinae granulata
aspergillus	Aspergillus auricularis
bacillus	Bacillus proteus
bacteroides	Bacteroides fragilis
borrelia	Borrelia hispanica
campylobacter	Campylobacter fetus
candida	Candida albicans
cellvibrio	Cellvibrio fulvus
chromobacterium	Chromobacterium amythistinum
clostridium	Clostridium difficile
corynebacterium	Corynebacterium hoagii
cysticercus	Cysticercus ovis
diplococcus	Diplococcus pneumoniae
echinostoma	Echinostoma melis
endomyces	Endomyces capsulatus
entamoeba	Entamoeba tropicalis
enterobacter	Enterobacter cloacae
escherichia	Escherichia coli
filaria	Filaria labialis
hemophilus	Hemophilus influenzae
hermodendrum	Hermodendrum rossicum
klebsiella	Klebsiella oxytoca
lactobacillus	Lactobacillus fermenti
microsporum	Microsporum fulvum
monilia	Monilia sitophila
mycobacterium	Mycobacterium microti
mycoplasma	Mycoplasma buccale
neisseria	Neisseria mucosa
peptococcus	Peptococcus magnus
proteus	Proteus filamenta
pseudomonas	Pseudomonas aeruginosa
saccharomyces	Saccharomyces capillitii
salmonella	Salmonella typhosa
serratia	Serratia indica
shigella	Shigella dysenteriae
staphylococcus	Staph aureus
streptococcus	Strep pneumoniae
saenia	Taenia lata
seponema	Treponema orale
trichomonas	Trichomonas vaginalis

Figure 14–1   Common genus/species and family names of diseases

          iii. hand
          iv. foot
        b. spine
      B. Objective
        1. Vomiting
        2. Diarrhea
    II. Not so common symptoms
      A. Thrombosis
      B. Hemorrhage
      C. Cyanosis

14. Capitalize **trade names** or **brand names** (names that are registered trademarks or officially contain the registered trademark symbol ® in their names) of drugs and other words. (Consult the *PDR* or a drug index for further information about brand versus generic drug names.)

    Examples: The discharge medications were: Dyazide, hydrochlorothiazide, aspirin, Tylenol, erythromycin and Maalox.
           Motrin is a brand name for ibuprofen.
           She is to take Pen-Vee K twice a day for two weeks.
           She should use Kleenex tissues and Vaseline petroleum jelly, and she should refrain from the use of Q-Tips.
           The trade name Xerox should not be interchanged with terms for the process of photostatic copying.

14–B General Rules for Word Capitalization in Medical Transcription

1. Rules for capitalizing headings and subheadings:
In general, capitalize the entire word with a formal subject heading and capitalize only the first letters of all words in a subheading. Capitalize only the first letter of the first word of subheadings following a formal heading.

    Examples: HISTORY OF PRESENT ILLNESS: The patient is a 32-year-old . . .
           Family History: The patient's mother died at age 59 of a . . .
           PHYSICAL EXAMINATION: Vital signs: Temperature 100, pulse 80, respirations 24, and blood pressure 140/90.

For the basic six reports, use the following guide for the capitalization of headings and subheadings.

i. History and Physical Report
CHIEF COMPLAINT:
HISTORY OF PRESENT ILLNESS: (or, SUBJECTIVE:)
PAST HISTORY:
Past Medical History:
Family History:
Social History/Habits:
REVIEW OF SYSTEMS:
Skin:

Head, Eyes, Ears, Nose and Throat:
Mouth:
Neck:
Chest:
Lungs:
Heart:
Abdomen:
Extremities: (or, Musculoskeletal:)
Neurologic:
Other System Components:
PHYSICAL EXAMINATION: (or, OBJECTIVE:)
    (same subheadings as in Review of Systems)
LABORATORY DATA: ASSESSMENT: (or, DIAGNOSIS: or, IMPRESSION:)
PLAN:

  ii. Consultation Report
DATE OF CONSULTATION:
REASON FOR CONSULTATION:
(the primary data for the consultation needs no heading)
ASSESSMENT:
RECOMMENDATIONS:

 iii. Pathology Report
TISSUE SUBMITTED:
GROSS:
MICROSCOPIC:
IMPRESSION:

 iv. Operative Report
PREOPERATIVE DIAGNOSIS:
POSTOPERATIVE DIAGNOSIS:
OPERATION(S) PERFORMED:
FINDINGS AND PROCEDURE:
Sponge count:
Estimated blood loss:

  v. Radiology Report
(PROCEDURE NAME)   DATE:
IMPRESSION:

 vi. Discharge Summary
DATE OF ADMISSION:
DATE OF DISCHARGE:
ADMITTING DIAGNOSIS:
CONSULTATIONS:
PROCEDURES:
HISTORY:
Past History:
PHYSICAL EXAMINATION:
LABORATORY DATA:
HOSPITAL COURSE:
DISCHARGE DIAGNOSIS(ES):

2. With sentences describing patient allergies, key the entire sentence either in bold print or uppercase when the allergies are noted as part of the history.

Examples: **She is allergic to penicillin and codeine.** She has no other
complaints.

The patient is up to date on his immunizations. HE IS
ALLERGIC TO ASPIRIN.

3. Capitalize the introductory words "Whereas," Resolved," and "Therefore"
when keying corporate or meeting minutes, and capitalize the first letter of the
word immediately following the introductory word. (Some institutions capitalize only the first letter of the introductory words "Whereas", "Resolved",
and "Therefore" and leave the subsequent words lowercase.)

Examples   WHEREAS, The board of directors has voted to maximize
employee benefits.

RESOLVED, Profit-sharing will commence October 1.

THEREFORE, The motion passed.

4. Capitalize the title and subject headings in a memorandum, and capitalize the
reference line introducer in letter correspondence. (Some institutions capitalize
the entire reference line in letter correspondence.)

Examples:

MEMO

FROM:	Suman Jakarta, M.D.
TO:	Lab Technicians
RE:	Test Reporting Techniques
DATE:	June 21, XXXX

Malcolm Kenya, M.D.
20001 Peripheral Drive
Tacoma, Washington 98000
RE: Sally Saraguchi

5. Capitalize most abbreviations where the initials of the abbreviation stand for
separate words. With lowercase abbreviations, use periods between the letters.
Capitalize abbreviations used in geographical directions:

Examples: The CBC showed 7,900 WBCs and 300 RBCs.

Her rhinitis medicamentosa was treated with steroids p.r.n.

The patient's address was 15 S.E. Main Street.

14-C General Rules for Conditions in Which Capitalization Should Not Be Used

1. Do not capitalize names of relationships, unless they substitute for proper names.

Examples: The patient's aunt was present.

His mom was also quite helpful.

He remembered Father.

2. Do not capitalize names of hospital or medical departments, specialties, or
hospital rooms unless they include the entire hospital name.

Examples: The patient arrived via ambulance at the Mercy Hospital
Emergency Room, and she was taken to the intensive
care unit at that time.

Dr. Larry Hornton, orthopedist, performed a consultation.

The patient was sent for an ophthalmology evaluation.

3. Do not capitalize Greek letters.
    Examples: alpha

    beta-lactamase

    gamma rays
4. Do not capitalize some units of measure.
    Examples: There were 3 mg of fluid.

    The infant weighed 7 lb., 6 oz.

    The Discharge Summary took 2.5 megs of space.
    but
    The Discharge Summary took 2500 Kb of space.
5. Do not capitalize the abbreviations "a.m." or "p.m."
    Examples: The patient arrived to the ER at 12:00 p.m.

    She was placed on a regimen of a.m. diuretics.
6. Do not capitalize most abbreviations relating to medications.
    Examples: Take two tablets q.i.d. × 3 days.

    Take 10 tsp. at h.s. p.r.n.
7. Do not capitalize or abbreviate species name when expressed together with genus name, and do not capitalize the plural or adjectival form of a genus name.

Examples.	C. difficile	*not*	C. Difficile
	H. influenzae	*not*	H. flu
	staphylococci	*not*	Staphylococci
	streptococcal	*not*	Streptococcal

8. Do not capitalize quotations that are sentence dependent, whether they are sentence fragments or complete sentences.
    Examples: Dr. Smith said to schedule "no more patients on the 3rd of July."

    The operative permit implied that "the patient agrees to the procedure."

Summary of Concepts

- Capitalize the first letter of the first words of sentences, proper names and nouns, direct quotations, complete parenthetical sentences, salutations and complimentary closes, genus names and eponym in diseases, most Roman numerals, and brand and trade names.
- Capitalize the entire word with allergies, introductory words of corporate minutes, memorandum headings and most abbreviations.
- Become familiar with the rules for capitalization of medical report headings and subheadings.
- Do not capitalize names of relationships, informal names of hospital departments, Greek letters, some units of measure, a.m. or p.m. designations, most abbreviations relating to medicines, and sentence-dependent quotations.

Chapter 15

Plural and Possessive Forms

Overview: Plural and possessive forms are often confused. Many times a physician dictates the singular form of a word that should be plural, or he or she incorrectly pronounces the plural word or gives punctuation instructions that would make the word possessive. Following are some rules and aids for making words plural and possessive.

Key Words

adenomata

agenda

alumni

anuli

bacteria

calices

calyces

condylomata

cornua

criteria

diverticula

epididymides

fibromata

foramina

fundi

ganglia

genua

halluces

larvae

meninges

nares

petechiae

phenomena

plural

possessive

prostheses

semina

striae

velamina

ventricornua

15–A The Plural Form

In the English language, making words and phrases **plural** (a grammatical method of signifying that a word indicates more than one) is oftentimes accomplished simply by adding the letter "s" to the end of a word. However, it is not always that simple. If the word is a common noun and ends in the letter "y", for example, the plural form would be to drop the "y" and add the suffix "-ies". Always consult a medical dictionary regarding whether to make a medical term plural.

Some general rules for creating the plural form of a variety of words used in medical transcription follow.

15–B Plural Form Rules for American (English) Words

1. For most words, simply add "s".
    Examples: pill → pills
                  symptom → symptoms
                  ear → ears
2. For most words ending in "z", "s", "x", "ch" or "sh", add "es".
    Examples: search → searches
                  brush → brushes
                  gas → gases
3. For words ending in "y", if the "y" is preceded by a consonant, change the "y" to "i" and add "es".
    Examples: extremity → extremities
                  disparity → disparities
                  dichotomy → dichotomies
4. For words ending in "y", if the "y" is preceded by a vowel, add "s".
    Examples: key → keys
                  relay → relays
                  gurney → gurneys

15–C Plural Form Rules for Latin, Greek, or Latin- or Greek-based Words

Become familiar with the definitions of the plural words that follow.

1. For words ending in "x", change the "e" to "y" or the "i" to "y" if there is an "e" or "i" preceding the "x", and then change the "x" to "c" or "g" and add "es".
    Examples: calyx → **calyces** or **calices** (cuplike organs or cavities)
                  hallux → **halluces** (more than one great toe)
                  meninx → **meninges** (membranes)
2. For words ending in "a", keep the "a" and add "e".
    Examples: larva → **larvae** (developing forms of insects after they have emerged from eggs and before they transform into the pupal form)
                  petechia → **petechiae** (small, purple-colored, hemorrhagic spots)
                  stria → **striae** (lines or bands either elevated above or depressed below tissue surrounding them, or differing in color from each other)

3. For words ending in "is", drop the "is" and add "es" or "ides".

   Examples: epididymis → **epididymides** (more then one small oblong body lying on the posterior surface of the testes)

   naris → **nares** (nostrils of the nose)

   prosthesis → **prostheses** (artificial replacements of body parts or extremities)

4. For words ending in "um", drop the "um" and add "a".

   Examples: agendum → **agenda** (a plan, outline or listing of things to be done, especially in a meeting)

   bacterium → **bacteria** (microorganisms of the class Schizomycetes)

   diverticulum → **diverticula** (sacs or pouches in the organ walls)

5. For words ending in "us", drop the "us" and add "i" (notable exceptions are the words "virus" and "sinus", where you would add "es").

   Examples: alumnus → **alumni** (one or more persons who have attended or graduated from an educational institution)

   anulus → **anuli** (ring-shaped structures)

   fundus → **fundi** (more than one base portion or major body of a hollow organ)

6. For words ending in "en", drop the "en" and add "ina".

   Examples: foramen → **foramina** (orifices, openings or passages between structures)

   semen → **semina** (a collection of thick, opalescent, viscid secretion of the male discharged during sexual activity)

   velamen → **velamina** (covering membranes)

7. For words ending in "on", drop the "on" and add "a".

   Examples: criterion → **criteria** (characterizing traits or requirements)

   ganglion → **ganglia** (masses of nervous tissue)

   phenomenon → **phenomena** (facts or events able to be detected by the senses)

8. For words ending in "oma", change the "oma" to "omata".

   Examples: adenoma → **adenomata** (neoplasms of glandular epithelium)

   condyloma → **condylomata** (wartlike growths of genital or anorectal skin)

   fibroma → **fibromata** (fibrous, encapsulated connective tissue tumors)

9. For words ending in "u", change the "u" to "ua".

   Examples: cornu → **cornua** (hornlike projections)

   genu → **genua** (knees, or kneelike structures)

   ventricornu → **ventricornua** (more than one anterior ventral horn of the gray matter of the spinal cord)

15–D Special Rules for Plural Cases

1. For plurals of single letters, numbers, words named as words, or lowercase abbreviations, add an apostrophe + "s" (also drop the periods when making lowercase abbreviations plural).

   Examples: The surgery would be performed, there would be no if's, and's or but's.
   On speech evaluation, the patient had difficulty pronouncing his L's, R's and Th's.
   There are two 6's in 1966. Everyone knows the 1960's were wild.
   The patient could tolerate the n.p.o. diets, but he had trouble tolerating the po's.

2. For plurals of compound words that contain only equal nouns or nouns and verbs, make only the last word of the compound plural.

   Examples: There was one nurse practitioner present. → There were many nurse practitioners present.
   The patient had a breakthrough in his prophylaxis. → The patient had several breakthroughs in his prophylaxis.
   A cross-match was done of the child's blood. → Two cross-matches were done of the child's blood.

3. For plurals of compound words that contain unequal nouns or nouns with other parts of speech such as prepositions, make only the main noun of the compound plural.

   Examples: His mother-in-law was in group therapy. → The mothers-in-law were in group therapy.
   There was a teaspoonful of medicine in the dropper. → There were three teaspoonsful of medicine in the dropper.
   The accident would not have occurred at a speed of one mile-per-hour. → The accident occurred at a speed of 50 miles-per-hour.

4. Do not change abbreviated units of measure when making them plural.

   Examples: 1 mg of fluid → 191 mg of fluid
   1 lb. of adipose → 3 lb. of adipose
   1 oz. of plasma → 16 oz. of plasma

5. When it is necessary to write out units of measure, add an "s" to make the word plural.

   Examples: There were many millimeters of fluid withdrawn.
   The patient weighed several kilograms.

15–E The Possessive Form

The possessive form, or the grammatical method of signifying that a word shows ownership or possession, also presents some challenges to the medical transcriptionist. The **possessive** form shows possession or ownership of someone or something by someone or something else. This possession can be expressed either with a clause containing "of", or with an apostrophe or an apostrophe + "s". More specific rules follow.

15–F General Possessive Form Rules

1. To form the possessive of singular or plural nouns that do not end in "s", add an apostrophe + "s".

    Examples: The patient felt he was no one's relative.
    The children's fevers were high.
    The men's room is located at the end of the hall.

2. To form the possessive of singular nouns or names that end in "s", add an apostrophe + "s" (an exception to this rule is when a noun or name ends in an "s" or a "z" sound, when a noun or name has more than one "s" sound, or when a noun or name sounds like it is already plural, in these cases, add only an apostrophe).

    Examples: Mr. Jones's physician lives in Vermont.
    The calculus's edges were uneven.
    Mr. Martinez' daughter signed the consent form.
    ["Martinez" ends in a "z" sound.]
    The archaeologists thought they had found Ramses' tomb.
    ["Ramses" contains two "s" sounds.]
    It was without question Mr. Bowles' handwriting.
    ["Bowles" sounds like it is already plural.]

3. To form the possessive of plural nouns or names that end in "s", add only an apostrophe.

    Examples: The otolaryngologists' symposium lasted one week.
    The Joneses' daughter was out of town.
    The pain was of three days' duration.

4. To form the possessive of compound nouns or word groups, add an apostrophe + "s" to the last word.

    Examples: The queen's lady-in-waiting's birthday was yesterday.
    Accidentally the surgeon removed someone else's tonsils.
    The president-elect's finance troubles were typical.

5. If two or more words each individually show possession, add an apostrophe + "s" to each word.

    Examples: Maria's, John's and Philip's diagnoses were similar.
    The doctor's and nurse's courses were different but
    prepared each of them well.

6. If two or more words each show joint possession, add an apostrophe + "s" to the last word only.

    Examples: Invoices are the patient and the insurance company's
    responsibility.
    Jerry and Jean's task was to study for the American Red
    Cross exam.

Summary of Concepts

- To make most American (English) words plural, simply add the letter "s"; some English words become plural by adding "es" or by changing a consonant and adding "es".
- There are several rules for making Greek- or Latin-based words plural. These rules include: changing an "x" ending to "c" or "g", and adding "es"; keeping an "a" ending and adding an "e"; dropping an "is" ending and adding "es" or "ides"; dropping an "um" ending and adding an "a"; dropping an "us" ending and adding an "i"; dropping an "en" ending and adding an "ina"; dropping an "on" ending and adding an "a"; changing an "oma" ending to "omata"; and changing a "u" ending to "ua".
- To make single letters, numbers, words named as words, or lowercase abbreviations plural, add "'s".
- To make equal compound words plural, make the last word of the compound plural; to make unequal compound words plural, make the main noun of the compound plural.
- Do not change abbreviated units of measure when making them plural, and when writing out units of measure, add an "s" to make the word plural.
- To form the possessive form of words that do not end in "s", add an "'s", and to form the possessive form of words ending in "s", add either an apostrophe or an "'s".
- To form the possessive of compound words, add an "'s" to the last word.
- To make two or more words show individual possession, add an "'s" to each word.
- To make two or more words show joint possession, add an "'s" to the last word only.

Chapter 16

Numbers and Number Combinations

Overview: Should you begin a sentence with a numeral? Do you use figures or written numbers when expressing a patient's age? These questions can be difficult to answer if one is not adept in the use of numbers and number combinations. Decisions regarding whether to use Arabic numerals, Roman numerals, or written numbers must constantly be made by medical transcriptionists. Use this chapter as a guide.

Key Words

Apgar ratings

Arabic numerals

cardinal numbers

digits

military time

numerals

ordinal numbers

Roman numerals

round numbers

suture

visual acuity

written number expressions

16–A Some Notes on Numbers

Numbers and number combinations can present a challenge to the medical transcriptionist. Some documents, such as legal documents, minutes and other similar records, require **written number expressions** (numbers expressed as words, such as one-hundred fifteen-thousand and forty-two) of all numbers, including dates. Other documents, such as statistical or technical reports, contain only **digits** (numeric symbols, or the characters 0, 1, 2, 3, 4, 5, 6, 7, 8 and 9), also called **numerals.** The majority of medical transcription, however, contains a mixture of written number expressions and digits.

There are many rules to follow for correctly keying numbers, and some of these conventions conflict with other rules. When in doubt, use the rule most specific to the particular situation in which the numbers are used. Following are the most common rules for expressing numbers in medical transcription.

16–B General Rules for Number Expressions As Figures

1. Use figures for numbers greater than nine, and spell out numbers one through nine. (This rule is specific to transcribing medical records; the number "10" may be spelled out in other types of writing, and some medical institutions prefer 10 to be spelled out.)

   Examples: There were 100,000 platelets in the blood.
   A deciliter consists of 10 liters.
   The patient was in the hospital for five days.

2. Use a combination of figures and words to express numbers greater than 999,999.

   Examples: The event included 10 million people.
   The $5 billion deficit would be hard to overcome.
   Construction costs for the new wing of the hospital are
   around $200 million.

3. Use commas to separate thousands from hundreds with figures.

   Examples: There were 11,600 WBCs on the blood analysis.
   The pathologist found 210,000 platelets during the CBC.
   The white count was 8,900.

4. Always use figures with chronological ages. (This rule is specific to transcribing medical records; ages may be spelled out in other types of writing.)

   Examples: The patient was 25 years old.
   She was a well-developed 9-year-old child.
   The 1-month-old baby had a sister age 2.

5. Use figures with most abbreviations, units of measure, laboratory data and symbols.

   Examples: On CBC there were 5 bands, 35 lymphs, and the pH was 6.5.
   An incision was made 5 cm superior to the peritoneum.
   At 100 degrees Fahrenheit, the reaction should be
   50% completed.

6. Use zero in numerical figure form as a placeholder with decimals and for consistency in an expression. Use a negative indefinite pronoun when possible to substitute for zero in an expression.

   Examples: The patient was placed on Synthroid 0.25 mg.
   The normal range for myeloblasts is 0.3–5.0%.
   There were no eosinophils present.

7. Use fractions with quantities of age and English measure and decimals with quantities of metric measure. Also, use figures with measurements including height, weight, width, depth and/or length, or in expressions using an "×" to represent "times" or "by."

   Examples: She was a 9-⁵⁄₁₂-year-old, white female.

The jagged laceration was 2.5 cm in width × 3.5 cm in length.

The patient's weight was 125½ lb.

Several 4 × 4's were used in the building.

8. Use figures with positive and negative (+ and –) signs, ratios and chemical symbols.

Examples: The Babinski's reflex was 2+/3+ bilaterally.

The value was – 6.

Titers of 1:80 or greater can be significant.

The CO_2 value was greater than the H_2O value.

9. Use figures with blood pressure and temperature values.

Examples: His blood pressure was elevated at 160/90.

A temperature of 99 degrees Fahrenheit or greater would be found in a febrile patient.

The wind chill factor was 9 degrees below 0.

10. Use figures with most drug values, but spell out the numbers when using words to describe the frequency of a dosage less than 10. Be consistent in using either figures or spelling out numbers.

Examples: The patient was given 25 mEq of Micro-K and prednisone 250 mg q 8h. t.i.d. for 10 days.

She was also given 1 inch of Nitropaste every four hours.

He was to take the medication at a dosage of 400 mg one every 12 hours as needed.

Her mother was to take Dyazide 50 mg 2 capsules b.i.d. × 1 month.

11. Use figures with **suture** (surgical stitch) values, and include dashes and # signs.

Examples: The surgeon used 4-0 Prolene sutures.

The wound was repaired with #1 nylon.

The pins were held in place with #20 gauge sutures.

12. Use **Roman numerals** (I, II, III, IV, V, etc.) with cranial nerves, obstetrical history, electrocardiographic limb leads, types and factors, and cancer stages (see Figure 16–1 for use of Roman numerals).

Examples: Cranial nerves II through XII were intact, although cranial nerve VIII showed minor abnormal signs.

She was gravida III para II SAB I.

Limb leads II through V on the EKG were mis-placed.

The patient, who had type II hyperlipidemia, had a factor VIII drawn.

The carcinoma was stage II.

13. Use **Arabic numerals** (1, 2, 3, 4, 5, etc.), also called **cardinal numbers,** with vertebrae and disc spaces, cardiac murmur grades, electrocardiographic chest leads, cancer grades and **visual acuity** (testing of level of acuteness or clearness of vision from various distances).

Examples: There was a herniation at the L5-S1 level, and a fracture at C3.

Arabic Numeral	Roman Numeral
1	I
2	II
3	III
4	IV
5	V
6	VI
7	VII
8	VIII
9	IX
10	X
11	XI
12	XII
13	XIII
14	XIV
15	XV
16	XVI
17	XVII
18	XVIII
19	XIX
20	XX
30	XXX
40	XL
50	L
60	LX
70	LXX
80	LXXX
90	XC
100	C
200	CC
300	CCC
400	CD
500	D
600	DC
700	DCC
800	DCCC
900	CM
1000	M

Figure 16–1   Roman numerals

On cardiac examination, a grade 2/6 murmur was
auscultated.

The sarcoma was grade 2.

Vision in the left eye was 20/400 and in the right eye 20/60.

14. Use figures for **Apgar ratings** (neonatal testing of physical condition, including heart rate, respiration, muscular tone, stimuli response, and skin tone performed at one and five minutes after birth), and spell out the minutes at which
the test was done.

> *Examples:*   Although the infant was premature, Apgars were 6 and 8 at
> one and five minutes.
>
> The baby had an initial Apgar score of 1 for heart rate, 1 for
> respiratory effort, 2 for muscle tone, 2 for reflex response
> and 1 for color.

15. Use figures and commas when expressing the day and year in dates; it is common to write out the name of the month. Do not use commas when expressing
only the month and year. Use ordinals only when the day precedes the month.

> *Examples:*   The patient's birth date was March 21, 1977.
>
> The operation was performed in May 1965, according to the
> patient.
>
> She was admitted on the 12th of June, and she was
> discharged on July 29.

16. Use figures, a colon and a.m. or p.m. with standard units of time; use figures
and the word "hours" with military units of time; and use figures and o'clock
with positions of a clock to indicate direction or proximity to the poles (see
Figure 16–2 for **military time** conversion).

> *Examples:*   The operation was performed at 8:00 a.m.
>
> She was brought to the emergency room at 1400 hours
> yesterday.
>
> An incision was made at the 9 o'clock position.

17. Use figures to indicate more than one item in a series. Use periods following
the digits if using a paragraph form for each item in the series, and use a single
closing parenthesis if using a same-line form for each item in the series.

> *Examples:*   DISCHARGE DIAGNOSES:
> 1. Left lower lobe infiltrate
> 2. Pneumonia
> 3. Hypertension
> *or*
> OPERATIONS PERFORMED:
> 1. Lumbar diskectomy
> 2. Decompression of cervical disc space #4
> *or*
> The patient's case made the following impressions: 1)
> cervicodorsal strain; 2) cervicodorsal spasms; and 3)
> radiculitis, right arm.
> *or*
> ADMITTING DIAGNOSIS: Pleurisy and pulmonary edema

Standard Time	Military Time
12:00 A.M. (midnight, beginning of day)	0000 hours
1:00 A.M.	0100 hours
2:00 A.M.	0200 hours
3:00 A.M.	0300 hours
4:00 A.M.	0400 hours
5:00 A.M.	0500 hours
6:00 A.M.	0600 hours
7:00 A.M.	0700 hours
8:00 A.M.	0800 hours
9:00 A.M.	0900 hours
10:00 A.M.	1000 hours
11:00 A.M.	1100 hours
12:00 P.M. (noon)	1200 hours
1:00 P.M.	1300 hours
2:00 P.M.	1400 hours
3:00 P.M.	1500 hours
4:00 P.M.	1600 hours
5:00 P.M.	1700 hours
6:00 P.M.	1800 hours
7:00 P.M.	1900 hours
8:00 P.M.	2000 hours
9:00 P.M.	2100 hours
10:00 P.M.	2200 hours
11:00 P.M.	2300 hours
12:00 P.M. (midnight, end of day)	2400 hours

Figure 16–2 Military time conversion chart

16–C General Rules for Written Number Expressions

1. Use words for numbers that begin sentences.
   Examples: Ten percent Xylocaine was used for the operation.
   One hundred and twenty-five people were present at the symposium.
   Fifteen thousand colonies of bacteria were seen on culture.
2. When using several numbers together, either consistently spell them out or use figures.

Examples: Seventy-five people out of one hundred use this medication.
Complications can occur between three and seven days.
The patient will be seen in follow-up in 7 to 10 days.

3. Spell out fractions of less than one, but use figures with fractions greater than one.

Examples: The precipitate was decreased by one-half percent.
Of patients with this disease, two-thirds benefit from
    treatment.
His physician decreased the dosage by one-fourth.
The condition lasted for 2-1/2 days.

4. Spell out fractions when using the word "of" between the fraction and what it modifies; use figures for fractions when they are units of measure.

Examples: Less than one-third of all patients prefer this medication.
The syringe was filled with 1/2 cc of Xylocaine.

5. Spell out single-digit **ordinal numbers** (numerals ending in -st, -nd, -rd and -th, such as first, second, 11th and 12th) and use figures for double-digit ordinals. Use Roman numerals with ordinals if the number ordinarily takes a Roman numeral.

Examples: There were fractures of the fourth, fifth and sixth ribs.
The patient was in the 12th grade.
The VIIIth cranial nerve was suspicious for nystagmus.

6. Spell out at least one word in a series of numbers that ordinarily would all be styled as figures. If the second number is shorter in length when written, spell out the second number. However, use figures if required for a particular numeric expression. Also hyphenate figures series that cannot be spelled out, for example, in addresses.

Examples: There were 20 15-mm lacerations scattered on the upper dorsum of the nose. → There were twenty 15-mm lacerations scattered on the upper dorsum of the nose.
She found two one-half inch notes attached to the chart. → She found two ½-inch notes attached to the chart.
The physician assistant noted that the patient answered 45 12-part questions on the test. → The physician assistant noted that the patient answered 45 twelve-part questions on the test.
He lives at 1100-305th Street North.

7. **Round numbers,** numbers that end in zero or are approximate in value, especially those that can be written in one or two words, can be either spelled out or expressed as digits. In the context of text, such as in letters, chart notes, and so on, round numbers may be either spelled out or expressed as figures; in the context of data recording, such as in laboratory data, tables, and so on, round numbers should be expressed as figures.

Examples: The reimbursement was off by seven hundred dollars.
Over five thousand patients were included in the study.
LABORATORY DATA: The CBC showed 100,000 platelets.

Summary of Concepts

- Use numerals with expressions of numbers greater than nine, chronological ages, fractions that are greater than one or used as units of measure, and double-digit ordinals.
- Use figures with most abbreviations; with units of measure; with laboratory data and symbols; with height, width, weight, depth and length measurements; with positive and negative signs; with ratios and chemical symbols; with blood pressure and temperature values; with most drug values; with suture values; with Apgar scores; with days and years in dates; and with expressions of time.
- Use written numerical expressions to indicate the following numbers and number expressions: numbers less than or equal to nine, numbers that begin sentences, fractions less than one, numerical words used to describe frequency of a drug dosage less than 10, minutes at which Apgar testing is performed, single-digit ordinals, round or approximate numbers used in text (if preferred), and the month in dates.
- Become familiar with Roman numerals and the rules regarding them.
- Become familiar with military time and the rules regarding it.
- Know when to use a combination of figures and written expressions of words.

Chapter 17

Commonly Confused Words, Misspelled Words and Spelling Hints

Overview: English can be a very difficult language to master. Many errors in writing are related to spelling. As a medical transcriptionist, you will find that many words are often confused or misspelled. To maintain your employer's or client's quality standards, you must ensure that the words you use are correct. Confused words can be a special problem, as most spell-checking functions on word processing programs will not alert you to this. Misspelled words will be flagged, but if the word is acceptable, incorrectly used or not, it usually will go unnoticed until printed or proofread (or in the worst case scenario, sent to the employer or client) unless you are familiar with commonly confused words. Consistent use of a dictionary will provide the greatest help, although many spelling problems can be avoided by following a few rules. The following is a guide to spelling hints, commonly confused words and misspelled words.

Key Words

American spellings	consonant
annunciation	preferred usage
commonly confused words	pronunciation
commonly misspelled English words	syllable
commonly misspelled medical terms	vowel

17–A Commonly Confused Words

A list of **commonly confused words** follows. Each word listed has the potential to be confused with another word. Most of these words are homonyms and sound alike. Learn the differences in the meaning and spelling of each word, so when these words are encountered in dictation you will be prepared to make the correct choice.

abduct (to flex away) vs. *adduct* (to flex inward)

accept (to receive willingly) vs. *except* (excluding)

advice (n. an opinion) vs. *advise* (v. to give an opinion)

a febrile patient (a patient with fever) vs. *an afebrile* patient (a patient without fever)

affect (n. psychological disposition; or v. to change or influence) vs. *effect* (n. a result; or v. to cause or bring about change)

allusion (indirect or casual mention) vs. *elusion* (an evading of something) vs. *illusion* (misleading appearance)

anonymous (nameless or unidentified) vs. *unanimous* (unified, especially a vote)

ante- (before) vs. *anti-* (against)

anterior (pertaining to the front part) vs. *interior* (pertaining to the inside part) vs. *inferior* (pertaining to the lesser part)

arrhythmia (irregular heart rhythm) vs. *erythema* (redness, especially of the skin)

assure (to promise) vs. *ensure* (to guarantee) vs. *insure* (to provide insurance)

aural (pertaining to the ears) vs. *oral* (pertaining to the mouth)

carotene (a yellowish chemical pigment) vs. *keratin* (a protein found in teeth, skin and nails)

cella (an enclosure) vs. *sella* (a saddle)

censor (to edit) vs. *censure* (to reprimand)

cite (a notation) vs. *site* (location) vs. *sight* (vision)

climatic (pertaining to the weather) vs. *climactic* (pertaining to a climax)

coarse (thick) vs. *course* (a path or regimen)

complement (something that completes) vs. *compliment* (something that flatters or praises)

conscience (sense of moral standards, or sense of right and wrong) vs. *conscious* (state of being awake or alert)

cord (a thick string, such as the spinal cord) vs. *chord* (a string or group of strings that produces sound, such as piano chords)

cystalgic (pain the bladder) vs. *systolic* (pertaining to a cycle of the heart beat)

cytology (cell biology) vs. *sitology* (the study of dietetics)

decision (a choice) vs. *discission* (an incision)

defuse (to strain or make nonfunctional) vs. *diffuse* (spread out)

descent (going down) vs. *dissent* (to disagree)

discreet (careful or prudent) vs. *discrete* (unrelated)

ductal (pertaining to a channel) vs. *ductile* (flexible)

dysphagia (inability to eat or swallow) vs. *dysphasia* (inability to speak)

effected (produced a desired result) or *effect* (a result) vs. *affected* (influenced or emotionally moved) or *affect* (emotional condition)

elicit (bring forth) vs. *illicit* (unlawful)

emanate (come from) vs. *eminent* (prominent) vs. *imminent* (likely to happen)

enervation (weakening) vs. *innervation* (distribution of nerves) vs. *innovation* (new method)

explicit (distinct or not vague) vs. *implicit* (implied)

facial (having to do with the face) vs. *fascial* (having to do with fibrous tissue)

farther (an extra distance) vs. *further* (an additional amount; also)

Feldene (anti-arthritic medication) vs. *Seldane* (antihistamine medication)

flanges (dental edges or borders) vs. *phalanges* (fingers, toes or digital protrusion)

gauge (a measurement) vs. *gouge* (to scoop out)

idle (not active) vs. *idol* (symbol of worship)

ileum (intestine) vs. *ilium* (hip bone)

inter- (between) vs. *intra-* (within)

it's (contraction for it + is) vs. *its* (possessive pronoun for something belonging to it)

knuckle (dorsal aspect of the phalangeal joints) vs. *nuchal* (pertaining to the neck)

labile (not fixed or shifting) vs. *labial* (pertaining to the lips)

later (at a subsequent time) vs. *latter* (the second or more recent of two previously named items)

lay (to place or put, used with objects) vs. *lie* (to recline, used with subjects, to deceive)

led (past tense of the verb "to lead") vs. *lead* (present tense of the verb "to lead", or a chemical element)

liable (accountable) vs. *libel* (disparaging or defamatory comment)

lichen (plant formed from algae and fungus) vs. *liken* (to compare)

loop (a bend in a cordlike structure) vs. *loupe* (a magnifying lens)

loose (not tight) vs. *lose* (to misplace, to be defeated)

meiosis (cell division) vs. *miosis* (constriction of the pupils)

moral (a. ethical; n. lesson) vs. *morale* (attitude or mood)

mucous (adj., pertaining to mucus) vs. *mucus* (noun form of mucus)

osteal (bony) vs. *ostial* (pertaining to an opening into a tubular organ or between two body cavities)

packed (bundled) vs. *pact* (agreement)

palpation (examination by feeling with fingers) vs. *palpitation* (throbbing or arrhythmia)

paracytic (lying among cells) vs. *parasitic* (pertaining to a parasite)

passed (went by, dissipated, or cessation) vs. *past* (in a former time)

pediculous (lice-infested) vs. *pediculus* (a pedicle or stemlike structure)

penile (pertaining to the penis) vs. *penal* (referring to the law enforcement system)

perfusion (a pouring through) vs. *profusion* (an abundance)

perineal (pertaining to the pelvic floor) vs. *perennial* (lasting a year or two years) vs. *peritoneal* (pertaining to the serous membrane lining the abdominopelvic walls) vs. *peroneal* (pertaining to the outer side of the leg)

petal (leaflike part) vs. *pedal* (pertaining to the foot)

plain (simple or single) vs. *plane* (a flat surface or a three-dimensional object)

precede (come before) vs. *proceed* (follow, or funds from an event)

principal (primary or head) vs. *principle* (a rule or law)

prostate (gland at the base of the male bladder) vs. *prostrate* (to lie flat; to overcome)

psychosis (mental disorder) vs. *sycosis* (hair follicle inflammation) *pupal* (pertaining to the second stage of an insect) vs. *pupil* (pertaining to the eye)

radical (extreme) vs. *radicle* (a small root)

rational (reasonable or logical) vs. *rationale* (explanation or justification)

reflex (involuntary reaction) vs. *reflux* (backward or return flow)

regimen (any methodical system, such as diet or exercise) vs. *regiment* (section of an Army division or control with strict discipline) vs. *regime* (political or ruling system)

retrocolic (pertaining to the colon) vs. *retrocollic* (pertaining to the back of the neck)

right (n. direction opposite of left, a privilege; v. or adj. correct) vs. *write* (to compose or record)

root (embedded part, or cause) vs. *route* (path)

rye (a type of grain) vs. *wry* (twisted or bent)

sac (pouchlike part) vs. *sack* (bag)

saccharin (a calorie-free sweetener) vs. *saccharine* (pertaining to sugar)

sail (v. to navigate; n. an object used to control wind on a boat) vs. *sale* (n. the selling of goods)

scatoma (fecal matter in the colon) vs. *scotoma* (area of depressed vision in the visual field)

scirrhous (hard) vs. *scirrhus* (a carcinoma)

set (to place something somewhere, used with objects) vs. *sit* (to rest on the buttocks, used with subjects; to remain for a time)

stationary (immovable) vs. *stationery* (writing paper)

their (possessive pronoun meaning belonging to them) vs. *there* (a place not here) vs. *they're* (contraction for they + are)

then (at a past time) vs. *than* (a word used to compare items)

to (prep. indicates movement toward) vs. *too* (adv. also) vs. *two* (a number following or greater than one)

-trophic (relating to nutrition) vs. *-tropic* (denoting a change)

vesical (pertaining to the bladder) vs. *vesicle* (a small sac containing liquid, especially of the skin)

viscous (having a high degree of friction when rubbed; thick and syrupy) vs. *viscus* (any of the large organs of the abdominal cavity)

waive (to defer or relinquish) vs. *wave* (v. to swell; n. a hand greeting)

who's (a contraction for who + is) vs. *whose* (a possessive form of the pronoun who)

Xanax (a tranquilizing medication) vs. *Zantac* (a medication for the treatment of ulcers)

your (possessive form of the pronoun you) vs. *you're* (contraction for you + are) vs. *yore* (long ago)

17–B Commonly Misspelled Words

The words that follow are often misspelled. Commit to memory the correct spelling of each of these commonly misspelled English words and medical terms.

Commonly Misspelled English Words

absence	acknowledgment	acquaint
amateur	analyze	anonymous
apologize	approximately	argument
athletic	auxiliary	bankruptcy
brochure	calendar	category
commitment	committee	concede
congratulations	conscientious	consensus
copyright	criticism	criticize
embarrass	environment	equipped
exaggeration	explanation	familial
fascinate	February	fluctuate
foreign	foresee	fourth
fulfillment	grammar	height
incidentally	insistence	integration
itinerary	judgment	leisure
liaison	license	likelihood
livelihood	loneliness	maintenance
miniature	miscellaneous	mortgage
necessary	ninety	noticeable
occurred	parallel	possession
privilege	profited	quandary
quantity	questionnaire	receipt
receive	recommendation	referral
relevant	restaurant	sacrilegious
schedule	separate	similar
sufficient	superintendent	supersede
supposedly	transferred	unanimous
undoubtedly	utilization	

Commonly Misspelled Medical Terms

accommodation	aggravated	alveolar
anthelix	anulus	apparent
aphthous	apneic	appendiceal
ascites	asymmetrical	asymptomatic
auricle	auricular	auscultation
breathe	bruit	buccal
caudal	choana	cholesteatoma
claudication	commissure	compatible
condyle	curette	curvilinear
defervescence	deglutition	dependent
desiccated	diarrhea	diuresis
Dyazide	ecchymosis	emittance
emphysema	empiric	eosinophil
erythema	eschar	Escherichia
exquisite	extraocular	fascicular
fluctuance	fluorescent	funduscopic

Commonly Misspelled Medical Terms (*continued*)

gallop	guaiac	hemoptysis
hyoid	inguinal	in situ
intermittent	in toto	Kerley B lines
labyrinthine	laryngeal	lysis
malar	maneuver	meconium
mucus	normocephalic	nystagmus
ophthalmology	palpitation	paresis
paroxysmal	phlegm	phonate
piriform sinus	Pseudomonas	pterygium
purulent	rhabdomyosarcoma	rhinitis
rhythm	sequelae	serpiginous
sialadenitis	Sjogrin's disease	sphenoid
telangiectasia	tenacious	threshold
tic	tinnitus	vesicular

17–C Guidelines for Preferred Usage

It is acceptable to use some English words and word groups in a variety of ways. However, some words and word groups used frequently in medical dictation have preferred forms. Use of the preferred form is called **preferred usage.** Be sure to consult with the physician or facility for which you are transcribing before making extensive changes. The following is a list of some preferred forms of common phrases used in dictation.

Word/Word Group	Preferred Form
at all times	always
at the present time	now
at this point in time	like
be sure and	be sure to
could of	could have
due to the fact that	because, due to
for the purpose of	for
in order to	to
in regard to, in regards to, with regard to	regarding
in the event that	if, should
might of	might have
O.K., o.k.	okay
should of	should have
towards	toward
try and	try to
until such time as	until
would of	would have

17–D Spelling Hints

1. *Do not rely exclusively on pronunciation.* With the English language, **pronunciation** (how a word is spoken, or pronounced) of words is often an unreliable method of determining their spelling. Also, differences in **annunciation** (how a word is formally spoken, or announced by various speakers) add to confusion in terms of spelling. For example, if a word ends in a sound similar to "uff", different correct suffixes could exist, depending upon the word: <u>stuff</u> or <u>rough</u>. Also, words that look alike may not sound alike: <u>rough</u>, <u>through</u>, <u>dough</u> and <u>trough</u>.

2. *Do remember that there can be different forms of the same word.* Remember that homonyms are words that sound alike or are spelled alike but are different in meaning, and synonyms are words with the same meanings. If confused about the correct use or spelling of a word, consult a dictionary.

3. *Do use preferred,* ***American spellings.*** For example, use "color" instead of "colour" "theater" instead of "theatre," and "canceled" instead of "cancelled." Other spellings (British, for example) usually use additional letters and often can confuse someone who has difficulty with spelling techniques.

4. *Do know the difference between words with "ie" and "ei" spellings.* Words such as receive and relieve sound alike, but the "i" + "e" combination is spelled differently in each. Use this clue to aid in spelling: "I" before "e", except after "c", or when pronounced "ay" as in "neighbor" and "weigh."

    Examples: beli<u>e</u>ve
                   retri<u>e</u>ve
                   conc<u>ei</u>ve
                   fr<u>ei</u>ght

    Special note: There are several exceptions to the aforementioned clue. If you question a particular spelling with "ei" and "ie" combinations, consult a dictionary. Become familiar with the following major exceptions to the clue:

apartheid	being	caffeine	codeine
deity	either	Fahrenheit	feisty
fluorescein	foreign	forfeit	geiger
heifer	height	heir	heist
leisure	neither	protein	reveille
seismograph	seizure	sheik	Sheila
sleight of hand	sovereign	stein	weird

5. *Do know when to keep or drop the final "e".* Drop the "e" before adding "-able", "-ible", or "-ing" if the ending begins with a **vowel** (the letters "a", "e", "i", "o" and "u").

    Examples: advis<u>a</u>ble
                   forcib<u>le</u>
                   surmis<u>ing</u>

    Exception: The silent "e" is kept to avoid confusion with another word, to avoid mispronunciation, or after a soft "c" or "g" to keep the sound of the **consonant** (nonvowel letters) soft.

Examples: dy<u>ing</u> vs. dy<u>eing</u>   (avoids confusion)
sing<u>ing</u> vs. sing<u>eing</u>
notic<u>eable</u>

6. *Do know when to keep or drop the final "y".* Change the "y" to "i" when it follows a consonant when adding an ending.
Examples: hurry → hur<u>ries</u>
apply → app<u>lied</u>

7. *Do double consonants when adding an ending with single syllable words.* When a word has a single **syllable** (a separate unit of a stress sound in words), double the last consonant before adding the ending.
Examples: stop → sto<u>pp</u>ing
tan → ta<u>nn</u>ed

Exceptions to this rule:

Do not, in most cases, double the final consonant when two vowels or a vowel and another consonant precede the final consonant.
Examples: start → star<u>ting</u>
jump → jum<u>ped</u>

Do double the final consonant when a single vowel precedes the final consonant and the stress falls on the last syllable of a two-syllable or more word.
Examples: refer → refe<u>rr</u>al
begin → begi<u>nn</u>ing

However, do not double the final consonant when two vowels or a vowel and another consonant precede the final consonant, or when the stress falls on a syllable other than the last syllable in a two-syllable or more word.
Examples: referral → refe<u>rence</u>
committed → commi<u>tment</u>

Summary of Concepts

- Recognize the differences in the meaning and spelling of commonly confused words.
- Know the correct spelling for commonly misspelled English words.
- Know the correct spelling for commonly misspelled medical terms.
- Use the preferred forms of common English phrases.
- Do not rely exclusively on the pronunciation of a word for its spelling.
- Remember that there can be different forms of the same word.
- Use preferred, American spellings of words.
- Understand the difference between words with "ie" and "ei" spellings, and know the exceptions to the major rule for "ei"/"ie" words.
- Know when to drop the final "e" of a word.
- Recognize when to keep or drop the final "y" of a word.
- Double consonants when adding an ending with single-syllable words.

Part Four

Medical Transcription Skills

Chapter 18

Editing Medical Dictation and Transcription

Overview: As stated in Chapter 1, the successful and proficient medical transcriptionist must be well skilled in editing. The transcriptionist must not only know when editing is necessary, he or she must know precisely how to properly edit to not change the meaning or context of the original dictation. The transcriptionist must use any prescribed guidelines given by the dictator or employer as well as her or his own discretion regarding the proper place, time and manner in which to edit dictation. This chapter provides a brief editing guide.

Key Words

content editing	hard copy
content errors	proof
copy	proofreading
copyediting	spell checking
editing	syntax
edits	typesetting
flagging	typographical errors

18–A The Importance of Editing in Medical Transcription

Editing, as defined in Chapter 1, What Is Medical Transcription, is the assembling or reassembling of a word, group of words, or document by cutting, pasting, adding, deleting and rearranging. Further, editing is the process of integrating word usage, grammar, punctuation, correct spelling and other mechanics into dictation to make the transcription clear, concise and logical. Finally, editing is effectively transforming raw, draft-quality written material into final **hard copy**

(information written, typed or printed on paper) suitable for receiving signature and/or publication.

Because of the major importance of editing, a thorough knowledge of the techniques, guidelines and rules pertaining to editing medical dictation and transcription is essential if one endeavors to become a successful medical transcriptionist. Always keep in mind while editing medical dictation that each dictator has his or her own style and preference; consult the facility or dictator for whom you are working regarding how much and what type of editing the institution or individual dictator allows.

18–B The Steps of Editing

There are three steps involved in editing: 1) copyediting, 2) content editing, and 3) spell checking. **Copyediting** is literally editing the **copy** (typed or printed text or information) for **typographical errors** made by the transcriptionist in the format, arrangement and printing of typed data, also called "typos." **Content editing** is editing the copy for **content errors,** including errors in style, **syntax** (grammar and sentence structure) and punctuation, made either by the transcriptionist or the dictator. **Spell checking** is checking the spelling of a document either manually (with a dictionary or other reference material) or, more commonly, electronically, using a special feature of a computer word-processing program designed specifically for checking the spelling (but not confused words) of text within the document.

Literally, **proofreading** is reading a **proof** (typed or keyed copy) of a document before the final printing or **typesetting** (setting into stylized type) of the copy. Copyediting and content editing often are grouped together as part of the proofreading process. However, they are two separate but similar processes that must be performed before spell checking a particular document. Keep in mind that spell checking is never a substitute for proofreading.

While content editing (and spell checking to a limited extent) can be performed while transcribing dictation, copyediting must be performed at the conclusion of the transcription process, before printing out a hard copy of the document. It often is helpful for the medical transcriptionist to be able to edit content errors concerning grammar and punctuation in dictation during the transcription process. Until the transcriptionist is well skilled in editing, however, he or she may choose to do all editing after the initial transcription of the medical dictation.

18–C Proofreading Guidelines

Use the following guidelines as steps when copyediting and content editing medical transcription.

First, *save the document* as is. Then ask the following questions when transcribing or looking over the text of a medical document:

1. Is the proper format (layout) applied (chart note type, correspondence type, report type, etc.)? [See Chapters 5, 6 and 7 for formatting guidelines.]

2. Are terms properly used (check for synonyms, homonyms and other confused words, and proper roots, prefixes and suffixes, etc.)? [See Chapter 8 for word usage guidelines.]
3. Are there any syntax errors? [See Chapter 9 for syntax guidelines.]
4. Is the punctuation correct (correct placement of commas, semicolons, periods, etc.)? [See Chapter 10 for punctuation guidelines.]
5. Are compound words and hyphenation used properly? [See Chapter 11 for compound words/hyphenation guidelines.]
6. Are contractions avoided? [See Chapter 12 for guidelines.]
7. Are shortened word forms appropriately used? [See Chapter 12 for guidelines.]
8. Are the proper forms of abbreviations, capitalization, plural and possessive forms, and numbers used? [See Chapters 13, 14, 15 and 16 for guidelines.]
9. Have all words with uncertain spelling or meaning been looked up in reference material? [See Chapter 4 for reference material types.]
10. Are names (especially patients' and physicians' names) spelled correctly? [See Chapter 17 for spelling hints.]
11. Are there any logical inconsistencies (items that do not seem correct or consistent in terms of reasoning)?
12. Are there any medical inconsistencies (items that do not appear to be correct or consistent in a medical sense)?
13. Are there any sequential inconsistencies (items that do not appear to be correct in terms of chronological time or order of occurrence)?
14. Does the document reflect the best job that I, as a medical transcriptionist, can do?

After answering these questions and making changes (called **edits**), leaving blanks, or **flagging** (attaching a Post-It® note or colored tab to the specific area of the document containing a possible error) the report when necessary, immediately save the document once again. It is not only frustrating, but time-consuming to finish proofreading a document and then have something unforeseen happen to the document (such as the electricity failing), which would necessitate having to redo all of the proofreading corrections. (This hint seems obvious, but many transcriptionists overlook this simple yet important task.) After the document is proofread and saved, spell check the document. Then save the document once again before printing so all changes and corrections are retained.

18–D General Content Editing Rules

Rules for general content editing follow. When these situations are encountered, make changes in the transcribed report. Usually prior consultation with the dictator is not necessary when implementing editorial changes for the following reasons.

1. Edit dictation when it is grammatically incorrect.
   Examples: **Dictation:**   "Her mother and her are to follow up with either Dr. Smith or I in two days."

Transcription: <u>She and her mother</u> are to follow up with either Dr. Smith <u>or me</u> in two days.
("Her" is an objective pronoun. "She" should be used because the pronoun is part of the subject of the sentence. Also, the preposition "with" takes an objective pronoun "me", instead of the subjective pronoun "I".)

Dictation: "The disease which the patient had he was treated for."
Transcription: The patient was treated for the disease that he had.
(The word "which" introduces a nonrestrictive clause, while "that" introduces a restrictive clause, and the sentence contains a restrictive clause, as it cannot be removed and have the same meaning. Also, the sentence ends in a preposition, so the sentence should be rearranged so it will not end in a preposition.)

Dictation: "There was no signs of hemorrhages, exudates or erythema on exam."
Transcription: There were no signs of hemorrhages, exudates or erythema on exam.
("There was" should be used with singular objects. "There were" should be used with plural objects, or a combination of plural and singular objects.)

2. Edit dictation when it is unclear, ambiguous, or could result in a misreading or misunderstanding.

Examples: **Dictation:** "The patient had mild obstruction sitting in the chair."
Transcription: The patient had mild obstruction, while sitting in the chair.
(The dictated sentence implies that the patient's obstruction was actually sitting in the chair. The transcribed sentence clarifies that the mild obstruction occurred while the patient was sitting in the chair.)

Dictation: "I will see her back in two days for re-exam."
Transcription: I will see her again in two days for re-examination.
or
She will come back to the office in two days for re-examination.
(The dictated sentence is ambiguous, implying that the dictator will be examining the patient's spine, or back, in two days. The transcribed sentence clarifies the fact that the patient will be seen and re-examined again in two days. The dictation actually was dictated by an otolaryngologist, who would not typically be examining the patient's back or spine.)

Dictation: "Dr. Brown, the patient's primary care physician, was contacted after he had the myocardial infarction."

Transcription: Dr. Brown, the patient's primary care physician, was contacted after the patient had the myocardial infarction.

(The dictated sentence implies that Dr. Brown, the physician, had the myocardial infarction. In fact, from the context of the dictation, the patient actually had the heart attack. The transcribed sentence makes the sentence clearer.)

3. Edit dictation when there is a medical or logical inconsistency.

Examples: **Dictation:**   "Hemoglobin was 42.7 and hematocrit was 14.1."

Transcription: Hemoglobin was 14.1 and hematocrit was 42.7.

(The normal reference value range for hemoglobin is from 11.2 to 19.5 grams, and the normal reference value range for hematocrit is 35 to 54 ml [see Appendix E]. Although laboratory results are often well outside the normal reference value range, it seems obvious that the dictator has transposed the values, which has resulted in a medical inconsistency, thus should be changed or flagged ["flagging" a report is attaching a sticky-backed note or a colored tag to the printed report]. If unsure about whether or not the dictation should remain as stated, print out a copy of both transcribed reports, as directed in section 18–E #3.)

Dictation: "The cardiologist was consulted, as the patient had marked erythema on his EKG."

Transcription: The cardiologist was consulted, as the patient had marked arrhythmia on his EKG.

("Erythema" means redness or flushing of the skin or membrane. "Arrhythmia" means a variation from the normal rhythm of the heartbeat. An electrocardiogram measures electrical currents of the heart; therefore, the use of the word "erythema" would be a medical inconsistency, as erythema could not be measured or detected on an electrocardiogram. Again, if unsure about whether or not the dictation should be edited, print two copies, as directed in section 18–E #3.)

Dictation: "The patient was seen in December of this year."

Transcribed: The patient was seen in December of 1995.

(The above dictation was done in March of 1996. Since December of 1996 had not yet arrived when the dictation was dictated, it is illogical and incorrect to transcribe that the patient was seen in the future, as was dictated. The transcription should be changed to reflect what the dictator apparently intended to say. If you were uncertain about the year, yet you knew that what was dictated was incorrect, again, you could print out two copies of the transcribed report, as directed in section 18–E #3.)

18–E Circumstances in Which You Should Not Edit

Specific instances in which you should not edit follow. When these situations are encountered, either key the transcription as dictated and/or leave a blank space, flag the report, and consult the dictator or a supervisor before making editorial changes.

1. Do not edit dictation when there is an unclear inconsistency, or when you are not reasonably sure about how to make a correction.

> *Examples:*   **Dictation:** "She had thrombophlebitis of the left leg . . . ASSESSMENT: Thrombophlebitis, right leg."
> **Transcription:**   She had thrombophlebitis of the __ leg . . . ASSESSMENT: Thrombophlebitis, __ leg.
> (It is unclear to which leg the dictator is referring, as he mentions first the left leg, and then later on in the dictation, the right leg. Since it is not possible to know with certainty which leg is the correct one, a blank should be left with a note attached, describing the problem in the dictation.)
>
> **Dictation:**   "PERRL. The left pupil was slightly unreactive."
> **Transcription:**   [Same.]
> (This transcription should be flagged, but left as is. It appears to be inconsistent that the left eye could be both reactive [PERRL = pupils equal, round and reactive to light] and slightly unreactive. However, you cannot be sure about how to edit the dictation, thus it should be left as is and the inconsistency pointed out to the to dictator.)
>
> **Dictation:**   "The patient had a mucousy discharge."
> **Transcription:**   [Same.]
> (Although the spell checking function on the word processor identifies the word "mucousy" as being an unacceptable word, and upon looking up the word in the dictionary no listing can be found, the dictation should remain as is, because there is no acceptable way to correct the word without making a possible change in the meaning of the sentence.)

2. Do not edit dictation if you are unsure about the dictator's meaning.

> *Examples:*   **Dictation:**   "The patient had PE on exam of the chest and lungs."
> **Transcription:**   [Same.]
> (This transcription should be flagged, but left as is. You cannot be sure about which abbreviation the dictator is referring, as "PE" could stand for pulmonary edema or pleural

effusion of which either would be appropriate in an examination of the chest and lungs. Since you cannot be sure about the correct abbreviation, leave it as is and point out the fact that the abbreviation remains in the transcription to the dictator.)

Dictation: "He was a 25 pack-a-day smoker."
Transcription: He was a __ pack-a-day smoker.
(In this dictation, "25 pack-a-day" smoker seems to be a logical inconsistency. You cannot be sure, however, whether the dictator means the subject smoked 25 cigarettes a day or something else. Therefore, a blank should be left and the transcription should be flagged.)

Dictation: "A chest x-ray was within . . . (cut-off) . . . limits."
Transcription: A chest x-ray was within __ limits."
(You might assume that the dictator means to say "normal" where he is cut off, but you cannot be sure. Therefore, leave a blank and flag the transcription.)

3. Do not edit dictation if the editorial changes would alter the dictator's meaning or style.

> *Examples:*   **Dictation:**   "Chest and lungs clear. No obvious changes since last exam. Will see patient back two days postop."
> **Transcription:**   [Same.]
> (Changing the dictated sentence grammatically by inserting articles, subject and predicates would result in changing the dictator's style.)
>
> **Dictation:**   "By her history, the patient had been afflicted with depression throughout the majority of her life. With regard to her status of mental condition upon examination, she was at all times lucid in processes of thought and speech. She was admitted due to the fact that observation was a necessary requirement until such time as she was felt to be of little danger to herself."
> **Transcription:**   [Same.]
> (Although this dictation is obviously wordy and contains several examples of word groups that should be replaced with preferred forms [see Chapter 17], this type of dictation appears to be the dictator's personal style. Since changing every instance of wordiness in transcribing this report could result in altering the dictator's style or meaning, do not edit this type of dictation without prior discussion with the dictator or approval by a supervisor.)
>
> **Dictation:**   She will follow up with her primary care and myself in two weeks.
> **Transcription:**   [Same.]

(There are two instances of individual style in this dictated sentence. The first, "her primary care," probably refers to her primary care physician, but this dictator's style is to omit the word "physician", so leave the dictation as is. After consultation with the individual dictator, he or she may allow you to alter the transcription to contain the word "physician"; however, do not alter dictation such as this without prior approval by the dictator. Also, it is preferable to use the objective pronoun "me" at the end of the sentence instead of the reflexive pronoun "myself", but this dictator's style is to use reflexive pronouns, in this case to sound more formal. Again, do not alter this type of dictation without prior approval or discussion.)

18–F Special Notes on Editing

1. Always take into consideration the policies and preferences of the physician, hospital, or client when there is a question regarding whether or not to edit.
2. Always be prepared to support your editorial changes. When there might be a question about something you have edited, or the manner in which you have edited, supply copies of written documentation from the reference materials or sources you used in making the editorial changes.
3. If you are unsure about whether the physician or dictator would approve of an edit, enclose printed copies of both the transcription, as it was originally dictated, as well as the edited version of the transcription. Note on an attached, separate piece of paper where and why you made the edit.
4. Remember that certain dictators have specific individual styles, and the dictator may not want his or her personal style altered by a transcriptionist without prior discussion. If a physician, for instance, consistently dictates in sentence fragments, and this is obviously her or his style, do not correct the sentences by making them complete. Leave the transcription as dictated; if the physician wants corrections, he or she will send the document back with specified revisions.
5. Do not edit to reflect your own personal writing style. You are not the author of your transcription; you are simply the one who transforms spoken language into written language. Only edit for the reasons explained in sections 18–C and 18–D.
6. Always leave a blank in the transcription if you cannot understand or hear some part of a dictation, if you feel there is an error or inconsistency you cannot correct, of if the dictator is cut off in his or her dictation. Always note to the dictator, on a separate piece of paper, that you have indeed left a blank.
7. Always double check a dictator's spelling. Although as a courtesy to the transcriptionist the dictator may go to the trouble of spelling out a word, many times the spelling is incorrect. Always look up unfamiliar words and spellings.
8. Always keep in mind that just as all people differ, so do dictators. While some dictators may appreciate frequent and thorough editing, others may regard the

dictation as being "their creation" and may resent such intervention, regardless of the admirable intentions of the transcriptionist. Be prepared to work with such dictators, and realize that they are ultimately responsible for the content of their report, since their signatures affirm its quality, authenticity and accuracy. Remember that the role of the medical transcriptionist is to help transform the transcription into clear, concise and more logical expressions of the same information, without reflecting the personal style, views or attitude of herself or himself.

18–G Humor versus Respect in Editing

All medical transcriptionists are likely to encounter, at some time during their careers, a dictated or transcribed word, phrase or sentence that strikes them as being humorous or amusing. It is natural to chuckle in these instances and you may feel free to do so; always keep in mind, however, that the transcription of medical records is serious business, and the confidentiality, sensitivity and privacy of the patient and dictator must always be maintained. A few examples of some phrases the author has encountered in proofreading transcribed dictation follow. Hopefully, this will provide you with some amusement and help you realize that medical transcription is not only a somber profession, but at times it also can provide a source of comical diversion.

1. **Transcribed:** "She would be a candidate for hearing aids if she sewed the sides."
   (The transcriptionist misheard "sewed the sides," when in fact the dictator meant "so decides.")
2. **Transcribed:** "The patient had no stupus."
   (The transcriptionist misheard a nonexistent word "stupus"; the dictator actually said the word "stiffness".)
3. **Transcribed:** "I will be in contact with the patient following his road testing."
   (The transcriptionist mistook the words "his road testing" for simply "further nose testing.")
4. **Transcribed:** "The youngster still has food in his ears."
   (The transcriptionist mistook the word "food" for "fluid.")
5. **Transcribed:** "The patient complained of a beasting."
   (After listening to the tape, and spending several minutes consulting a dictionary in an attempt to find an entry for "beasting," it was discovered that the dictator had actually said "bee sting.")

Summary of Concepts

- The knowledge of editing techniques are of major importance to the medical transcriptionist.
- There are three steps involved in editing: 1) copyediting, 2) content editing, and 3) spell checking. Copyediting and content editing are two separate but similar processes that must be performed before spell checking a particular document.

- Proofreading guidelines associated with editing a medical document include checking the document for errors in format, word usage, sentence syntax, and punctuation; misuse of compound words and hyphenation; improper use of contractions and shortened word forms; incorrect usage of abbreviations, capitalization, numbers, and usage of plural and possessive forms; and errors in spelling.
- When content editing using the general content editing rules, make changes in the transcribed report without prior consultation with the dictator.
- When a question arises during the content editing process about whether or not to edit, consult with either the dictator or your supervisor.
- Become familiar with the "Special Notes on Editing" section in this chapter.
- Although incorrectly transcribed medical dictation is sometimes humorous, always maintain respect for the patient and physician.

Chapter 19

The Business of Medical Transcription

Overview: Once you have completed your studies and become a medical transcriptionist, exactly what will you do with your skills? Will you work in a hospital or a medical office? Will you work as an independent contractor? What kind of income can you expect? What are the future prospects for your chosen career? All of these questions must be answered to acquire a full understanding of the business of medical transcription.

Key Words

clinic/multispecialty medical office

day shift

demographic criteria

emergency medical services (EMS)

employees

evening shift

flexibility

fringe benefits

full time

governmentally defined geographical area

graveyard shift

health-care market

heliport

independent contractor

in-house

Levels 1, 2, 3, 4 and 5 trauma care centers

macros

MTs

night shift

paraprofessionals

part time

payroll

production pay basis

profit sharing

regular office hours

rural market

shift differential

SICs

specialty medical office

split shifts

standard work day

subcontractors

suburban market

suburbs

temp

templates

temporary employment agency

urban market

wage pay basis

withholding

19-A Pros and Cons of Medical Transcription Environments

As discussed in Chapter 1, the medical transcriptionist's work environment is important in determining how he or she will go about his or her duties; medical transcriptionists (**MTs**) work in hospital medical record departments, pathology departments and radiology departments, medical offices and clinics, medical transcription service offices, and they also work in their own homes.

Because of the immense variety of medical terminology the new transcriptionist encounters, as well as the minimal experience she or he has, it is often helpful for an individual new to the medical transcription profession to spend some time, at least six months or more, working outside of the home in a hospital, medical office or medical transcription service environment. Although many new transcriptionists are eager to start working independently at home as an outside contractor, and some percentage of new MTs do go on to do so soon after completing their medical transcription education, the benefits of being in close proximity to other transcriptionists with more experience and knowledge of medical terms and pronunciations may outweigh the advantages of working out of one's own home.

There are several benefits and disadvantages to each working environment. These pros and cons will be discussed next.

The Hospital MT Environment In a hospital setting an MT becomes familiar with a wide variety of medical report transcription. This is the best setting in which to become well skilled in transcription of the "basic four." However, an MT working in a hospital will receive little or no experience in transcribing medical chart notes and letter correspondence, thus will not acquire as much specialized terminology experience as he or she would when working in a medical office. Usually the new MT will find several other transcriptionists working in the hospital from whom they will be able to receive additional help with terminology, pronunciations, facility formats and guidelines, and so on.

There is less **flexibility** (potential for movement or change) with work hours in a hospital medical transcription environment; a hospital MT usually must work a **standard work day,** eight hours a day, five days a week, and those hours usually remain the same week in and week out. Although all MTs, at least from time to time, will find themselves working on weekends, holidays and evening shifts, hospital MTs as a rule do not need a schedule as flexible as other MTs. Often, working a hospital-type schedule works best for MTs whose spouses or children have a set schedule that must be followed, for MTs who need consistent time off for travel or military service, and for MTs who need more of a set, consistent income.

Because they are **employees** (people who work directly for a facility with supervision, with set hours, and an outside-the-home working environment), hospitals place MTs on the **payroll** (an employer's list of employees entitled to pay, and the amounts due those employees) and usually pay their transcriptionists on a **wage pay basis** (pay in wages, based by the hour, day, week, month or year). This type of pay basis can be helpful for a new MT, since the speed at which the transcription is performed is less critical than in other settings, although, as in all settings, accuracy is always important. When an MT works as an employee in a hospital setting, for example, **fringe benefits** such as health and life insurance, paid vacations, and other incentives (such as retirement and pension plans) are often offered when the transcriptionist works **full time** (32 to 40 hours per week). Also, since the MT is an employee, taxes, Social Security, unemployment insurance, workers' compensation, and other payments are contributed by the employer and/or partially or entirely deducted from the employee's pay. Hospital MTs will likely be paid twice monthly, and pay raises are sometimes given to MTs on a yearly or twice-yearly basis. Also, special wage incentives are often given for those employees who work shifts other than during the regular business hours of 9:00 A.M. to 5:00 P.M., called a **shift differential.**

The Medical Office MT Environment   In a medical office setting, if the office is a specialty physician's office (such as a gastroenterologist, an otolaryngologist, etc.), the MT will likely become familiar with specialized medical terms specific to that specialty. In the **specialty medical office** environment the MT will not gain much experience in transcribing the "basic four" and will not be exposed to the wide variety of terminology involved in multispecialty transcription settings. Also, an MT working in a specialty medical office may be the only transcriptionist working in the clinic and will likely not have very much interaction with other MTs.

Like the hospital environment, medical office MTs usually do not have much flexibility in terms of work hours. In fact, the schedule of a medical office MT may require even more of a regimen, because most MTs who work in this environment usually keep the same schedule as the office, typically **regular office hours** (basically a 9:00 to 5:00 workday), although some medical office MTs work only **part time** (less than 32 hours per week). The medical office setting, like the hospital, is also a good working environment for those who need a set work schedule.

Similar to the hospital setting, the MT working in a medical office usually is an employee and is paid on a salaried or hourly basis, which can be beneficial to a new MT, again, when the speed at which the dictation is transcribed is important but less critical than the accuracy. These MTs often receive benefits, are subject to payroll deductions, and are paid vacation time similar to hospital MTs. Sometimes medical office MTs have the opportunity to participate in **profit sharing,** where portions of the profit from the medical practice are shared between the company and its employees.

The Medical Clinic/Multispecialty Medical Office MT Environment   In the **clinic/ multispecialty medical office** environment, an MT probably will spend the majority of time transcribing office chart notes, procedure notes and letter correspondence. Unlike working in the specialty physician's office, the MT will likely not encounter as much specialized terminology but will be exposed to a wide variety of general and systemic medical terminology. The MT may not have much exposure to the "basic four" in the clinic/multispecialty medical office. A larger clinic or multispecialty office, however, may employ several transcriptionists, and it is possible for a new MT to interact with other, perhaps more experienced, MTs.

Multispecialty clinic MTs usually have more flexibility in their environments than in the previously described work settings. Sometimes MTs working in clinics with large medical offices can go in to perform their work before or after regular business hours, and sometimes they can take advantage of taking work home with them if they have their own equipment. Some full-time MTs can work four 10-hour days, or three 12-hour days, instead of the typical five 8-hour days. Working **split shifts** (work shifts where the shifts are not eight continuous hours but are split throughout the day, such as between two employees each working a four-hour shift, one employee working a day shift and partial night shift, three employees sharing a nine-hour shift, etc.) can sometimes be an option for these MTs; other possibilities for flexible scheduling may also exist in the medical transcription department, however, because of this greater flexibility, the volume of work, consistency of the number of hours worked, and the resulting pay may be somewhat less predictable.

Like in the hospital and single-specialty medical office environments, the MT working in a multispecialty clinic is usually an employee and is most often paid on a wage basis, which, again, may be more beneficial for a new MT, or a combination wage/incentive program, where the employee is guaranteed a certain hourly rate plus may be eligible to receive incentive production pay. Vacations in this setting may or may not be paid or scheduled within consecutively occurring days. Multispecialty clinic MTs often receive benefits and paid vacation time and incur payroll deductions similar to the MTs mentioned previously, but these MTs often do not have the opportunity to partake in profit sharing.

The Medical Transcription Service MT Environment   At a medical transcription service, an MT probably will encounter just about every type of medical dictation, from the "basic six," including radiology and pathology reports, to medical office chart notes. Larger medical transcription services that employ **in-house** (working at the office site) MTs will likely have a large number of transcriptionists with whom a new MT can interact. However, most medical transcription services prefer that their MTs have a good deal more experience than those employed in other settings because of the larger variety of medical dictation the MT will encounter.

Some medical transcription services also employ MTs who work in their own home as **subcontractors** (non-employees who set their own work hours, work outside of the office, and have no direct supervision). Although most medical transcription services pay their transcription employees on a **production pay basis** (paid by the piece, or by how much is produced, usually in increments of lines, words, characters or keystrokes per hour), some pay on a wage basis. (Figure 19–1 illustrates a production rate conversion table.) Many MT services will also have customized medical transcription word-processing software programs, **templates** (shells of documents frequently used in which section headings, formats, etc., are saved and used as a shell for other new documents), **macros** (shortened word forms or abbreviations that stand for longer words, paragraphs, long sections of text or formatting codes that are frequently keyed and can be activated or played with the touch of one or two keys), and other computerized devices that can result in faster production and increased pay.

(All amounts are approximate only; actual income varies according to typing speed, skill level, accuracy, and actual production speed.)

If you are paid this per line (in cents)	And your approximate typing speed in words per minute (WPM) is . . .	Your production speed in lines per hour (LPH) should average . . .	Your hourly income in dollars per hour (hourly wage) should average . . .	Your yearly income working part time (4 hrs./day @ 1040 hrs./yr.) in dollars per year should average . . .	And your yearly income working full time (8 hrs./day @ 2080 hrs./yr.) should average . . .
6	40	80	$4.80	$4,992.00	$9,984.00
	60	120	7.20	7,488.00	14,976.00
	80	160	9.60	9,984.00	19,968.00
	100	200	12.00	12,480.00	24,960.00
9	40	80	7.20	7,488.00	14,688.00
	60	120	10.80	11,232.00	22,464.00
	80	160	14.40	14,976.00	29,952.00
	100	200	18.00	18,720.00	37,440.00
12	40	80	9.60	9,984.00	19,968.00
	60	120	14.40	14,976.00	29,952.00
	80	160	19.20	19,968.00	39,936.00
	100	200	24.00	24,960.00	49,920.00
15	40	80	12.00	12,480.00	24,960.00
	60	120	18.00	18,720.00	37,440.00
	80	160	24.00	24,960.00	49,920.00
	100	200	30.00	31,200.00	62,400.00

Figure 19–1   Production rate conversion table

The medical transcription service, out of all the out-of-home medical transcription environments, tends to employ or contract the fastest, most accurate transcriptionists, and service MTs usually have at least two years of general medical transcription experience. This environment has a lot to offer those MTs who do well without supervision, who have varied experience, who can maintain a high production rate over periods of time, and who need great flexibility in their work schedules but who do not yet have enough experience to be totally based at home.

Medical transcriptionists who work for transcription services may or may not receive fringe benefits or paid sick leave and time off. They also do not typically take part in profit sharing. Their work schedules are usually fairly liberal and flexible; however, because service MTs are more often paid on a production basis, and because the time worked per pay period often varies, many MTs who work for transcription services often find that their pay can vary somewhat from paycheck to paycheck (for example, an MT could work 40 hours one week and 35 hours the next, doing the same amount of work and receiving the same amount of pay, or could work 45 hours one week and 30 hours the next and receive a substantial difference in pay). Transcriptionists who work for services usually have their choice of working during the **day shift,** working morning hours, typically 7:00 A.M. to 3:00 P.M.; the **evening shift,** working evening hours, typically 3:00 P.M. to 11:00 P.M.; the **night shift** (also called the late shift, the overnight shift, or the **graveyard shift**), working night hours, typically 11:00 P.M. to 7:00 A.M.; or some other combination of hours and shifts. Shift workers often will receive a shift differential for working hours other than the day shift. Shift-working MTs also usually work a combination of weekday and weekend shifts.

Transcription service MTs usually are paid on a production basis and either fill out time cards or submit to the service the number of hours worked, lines keyed, and so on. These MTs are paid twice monthly or monthly. Subcontractor MTs usually are responsible for their own **withholding** (taking tax, usually federal income tax, amounts out of a paycheck and forwarding the amounts to governmental revenue departments) deductions and are sometimes required to make quarterly estimated tax payments.

Another environment similar to the medical transcription service, but usually not solely based on the medical transcription profession, is the **temporary employment agency.** Like the medical transcription service, a temporary employment agency contracts medical facilities and other clients, and the MT does not work directly for those clients but for the agency instead. Employment-related issues are directed to the agency instead of the facility at which the employee physically works. Potential employees are usually well screened by the agency in terms of education and experience before they are placed in a temporary position. National agencies such as Kelly, Norrell and Talent Tree supply temporary medical transcription and other workers to hospitals, medical offices and clinics.

The MT who works for such an agency is usually a temporary employee (called a **temp**) and works for a variety of facilities during his or her term of employment with the temporary agency. The pay is usually hourly, benefits may or may not be offered, and taxes and deductions will be withheld. As in the medical transcription service setting, the MT who is skilled in a variety of medical disciplines can expect to be paid more than other MTs. Well-skilled new medical transcriptionists may also find that temporary agencies are good potential employers, since a large variety of settings (and terminology) can be explored without making a commitment to one single work environment, facility or medical specialty.

The Home-Based MT Environment   The home-based medical transcriptionist has the greatest flexibility but also has much more responsibility. Home-based MTs, whether they work as subcontractors for larger services or directly for a physician's office, clinic or hospital, must have a full command of both general and specialty medical terminology and must build and maintain over the years their own medical reference library. (See Chapter 4 for tips on building a medical reference library.)

Home-based MTs can set their own work schedule (usually whatever hours they prefer to work within the limitations of the turnaround time), can often choose the amount of work they would like, and can oftentimes choose the type of dictator for whom they would like to transcribe before they start working with a particular account. These MTs also have the ability to choose their own work environments, hours and earning potential. Home-based MTs do not usually have to deal with the common stresses of working outside of the home, such as baby-sitting/child care, traffic, business attire, office politics, and overbearing supervisors. Home-based MTs also do not need to have a specific time of day or a specific amount of time set aside for taking lunch and breaks; they can schedule their work, break, meal and entertainment times whenever they choose within the time frame of meeting their deadlines.

If the home-based MT is a subcontractor for a larger service, he or she must submit to certain guidelines established by that service including, but not limited to, accuracy standards, production rates, volume of work done per pay period, billable amounts (e.g., if a line is a 50-space or a 60-space line), and turnaround time. If a home-based transcriptionist is an **independent contractor** (one who works alone directly for a physician, allied health clinician or other medical facility, with or without forming a business entity), he or she has a tremendous amount of responsibility, including marketing potential clients, contracting new clients, billing current clients, bookkeeping, collecting past due amounts when necessary, meeting turnaround times (even, sometimes, in inclement weather, in the face of transportation problems, or in other less-than-optimum conditions), and maintaining records and a large reference library.

Home-based MTs can rarely take time off, and when they do get vacation or sick time away from work it is almost never paid.

The home-based MT usually is either paid on a production basis or bills the client directly for transcription completed, on a monthly or twice-monthly basis. A few home-based MTs are paid hourly, but since this is a less accurate means of paying for services rendered most MTs working out of the home tend to be paid on a production scale.

The home-based MT is ultimately responsible for all facets of medical transcription he or she produces, including speed, turnaround, accuracy and price. The home-based MT must have a higher level of self-discipline, skill and management techniques than other MTs and also is usually responsible for his or her own withholding and deductions.

Some environments will undoubtedly present less of a stress factor for someone just entering the field of medical transcription, while other environments will provide more income and more flexibility than others. It is necessary that each new transcriptionist evaluate each medical transcription environment thoroughly, weighing the pros and cons of each, when making the decision regarding his or her ideal place in the world of medical transcription.

19–B Health-Care Markets

Just as there are various medical transcription environments in which a medical transcriptionist can work, there are various health-care markets in which an MT can work. These markets help determine what medical transcriptionists can expect to earn in the area in which they live and/or work. For medical transcription purposes, a **health-care market** encompasses a particular **governmentally defined geographical area** (an area with boundaries such as village, town, city, metropolitan area, county, state or region) along with certain **demographic criteria** (aspects related to the population in an area such as density, distribution and other characteristics like age) used to assess the level of medical care (determined by the number of available trauma care centers) necessary for the residents of that geographical area.

In terms of opportunity for medical transcription work, there are three basic health-care markets: 1) the urban market, 2) the suburban market, and 3) the rural market. These will be discussed next.

The Urban Market   The **urban market** is composed of a major city or metropolitan area. There are usually several major hospitals, single- and multispecialty clinics, and medical offices of physicians and **paraprofessionals** (allied medical professionals including physical therapists, massage therapists, chiropractors, psychologists, physician's assistants, nurse practitioners, and others who render some type of medical care).

The Suburban Market   The **suburban market** is composed of **suburbs** (outlying regions of a large city) including smaller cities, towns or other geographical areas surrounding an urban area. A suburban market can include one or more cities or towns, unincorporated county areas, or other natural geographical regions (such as homes located on a lake or in a mountain community). This market may contain one or more smaller hospitals (often called regional or community hospitals), a smaller number of clinics, and fewer offices of physicians and paraprofessionals than the urban market.

The Rural Market   The **rural market** includes most rural areas of a geographical region including farm areas, areas with smaller populations, and rustic areas located some distance from cities. Rural areas historically have been referred to as "country" areas. There may be one small hospital or no hospital at all, few, if any, clinics, a small number of physicians' offices, and no paraprofessionals. A rural market often has a physician or paraprofessional who only works in the area on a part-time, on-call or as-needed (p.r.n.) basis.

19–C Health-Care Market Levels of Care

For any particular population segment of a health-care market, there usually are a certain number of trauma care centers available to the public for the medical care of that population. These trauma care centers typically are hospitals that operate 24 hours a day, 365 days a year, but they now also include other more clinic-like settings including basic health-care and urgent health-care centers (operating more limited days and hours) within the health-care market. Every trauma care center must be able to provide **emergency medical services** (EMS). These include the assessment of the nature (triage) of and basic treatment of an injury, illness, or other circumstance requiring immediate medical attention. Usually, the larger the market the more and higher-level EMS and trauma centers are available to the population of that market.

Trauma care centers are divided into five categories: Level 1, Level 2, Level 3, Level 4 and Level 5, which will be discussed next.

A **Level 1 trauma care center** is the most comprehensive type of care center. Usually a major hospital, a Level 1 trauma care center must: 1) be capable of handling any and all types of basic, moderate, or critical care EMS (major injuries such as gun shot wounds, amputations, etc.; for casualties of major disasters such as earthquakes, fires, etc.; for major illnesses such as life-threatening cardiac, neurologic, circulatory problems, etc.); 2) possess on-site or nearby all currently available medical technological equipment (CT scans, MRIs, cardiopulmonary life-support systems, laboratory equipment, etc.); 3) be able to accept patients from all areas with lower level trauma care centers (such as via helicopter, ambulance, etc.); and 4) have on staff physicians who can provide care to patients in all medical specialties (such as cardiothoracic physicians and surgeons, neurologists and neurosurgeons, radiologists, pathologists, emergency room physicians, etc.) at high, moderate and low levels of care. Usually large urban markets have one or more Level 1 trauma care centers.

A **Level 2 trauma care center** is able to provide somewhat less care than the Level 1 trauma center. Usually a large hospital in an urban market, a Level 2 trauma care center can handle most types of critical medical emergencies and provide EMS for most severe major injuries, multiple-victim disaster casualties, and almost all major illnesses. A Level 2 trauma care center has a limited number of high-technology medical equipment such as CT scans or MRIs. It usually can accept patients arriving by both air and ground. A Level 2 trauma care center has most but not every type of medical specialty physician, either on staff or those who have admitting privileges.

Located in a suburban market, a **Level 3 trauma care center** is able to provide somewhat less care than a Level 2 trauma center. A Level 3 trauma care center is a hospital that can handle most types of critical medical emergencies but only provide limited care for very severe major injuries, very large numbers of victims concurrently in an emergency setting, or extensive major illnesses. Level 3 trauma care centers have few if any types of high-tech medical equipment such as CT scans or MRIs. A Level 3 trauma care center can accept patients arriving by ground transportation but may not have a **heliport** (a landing facility for a helicopter). It has on staff or on referral most major medical specialty physicians (cardiologists, neurologists, etc.) but may or may not have a great deal of surgical and highly specialized physicians always available.

Usually a hospital located in a very small suburban or rural market, a **Level 4 trauma care center** provides a lower level of care than a Level 3 trauma center. A Level 4 trauma care center can handle many types of critical medical emergencies but usually cannot provide long-term or comprehensive care for severe major injuries, multiple victim casualties, or major illnesses requiring highly specialized care. Level 4 trauma care centers usually have few if any types of high-tech medical equipment such as CT scans or MRIs. A Level 4 trauma care center can usually only accept patients arriving by ground transportation. It has on staff or on referral a few major medical specialty physicians (cardiologists, neurologists, etc.) and may have no surgical or highly specialized physicians available.

Located in a rural market, a **Level 5 trauma care center** provides a lower level of care than a Level 4 trauma center. Governmental (city, county, etc.) EMS units usually are not dispatched to Level 4 or 5 trauma centers. Usually Level 5 trauma care centers can provide only basic life-sustaining treatment for life-threatening injuries and illnesses. They normally are not equipped to handle multiple casualties. A Level 5 trauma care center may not be a hospital at all but merely a clinic or an office with a physician who is on call and trained in emergency medicine. A Level 5 trauma care center has only limited basic medical equipment on hand (it sometimes cannot provide such basic services as taking x-rays). A Level 5 trauma care center usually can only accept patients arriving by ground transportation. It generally has only one or two physicians on staff and usually must refer patients to a larger-level trauma care center for anything more than basic emergency services.

19–D How Health-Care Markets Affect Medical Transcription Pay

Since the opportunities for procuring medical transcription work increase proportionately with the size of the health-care market and the levels of trauma care centers within that market, the pay a medical transcriptionist receives also increases with the larger market (see Figure 19–2).

On the average, a production-paid MT who lives and works in a large urban area can expect to earn two to three times more than an MT who lives and works in a rural area. While an MT who transcribes for a Level 1 trauma care center will likely be paid more than an MT who transcribes for a Level 5 trauma care center, these are not set rules and pay varies from specific location to location. As a rule, where costs of living are higher (for example, on the East Coast in large metropolitan areas), the pay usually is higher. However, it would not be unheard of for a small rural general practitioner's medical transcriptionist to earn the same amount as a Level 1 or 2 trauma care center MT. Also keep in mind that with remote dictation and transcription an MT who lives in the country does not necessarily need to work in that market and vice versa.

19–E The Future of Medical Transcription

Medical transcription has made significant strides since AAMT, the first professional medical transcription organization, was formed in the mid-1970s. At that time, the approximately 1,000 or so actual medical transcriptionists were simply called "clerks" and were not thought of as trained professionals who were an integral part of the allied health care team (although many employers even in present times classify MT positions with "clerical/administrative" positions, most facilities realize that MTs are skilled, trained, often credentialed members of the workforce). (See Figure 19–3.)

The late 1990s saw the number of employee, subcontractor, and independent medical transcriptionists rise to more than 50,000, with specific medical

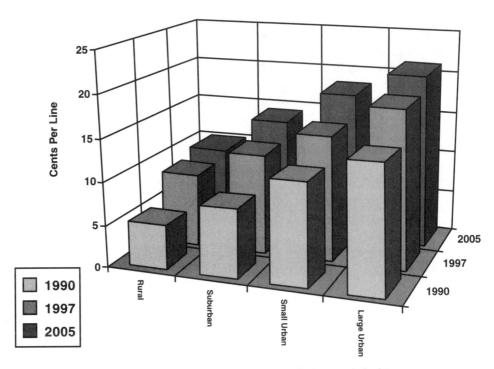

Figure 19–2   Approximate average production rates for medical transcriptionists

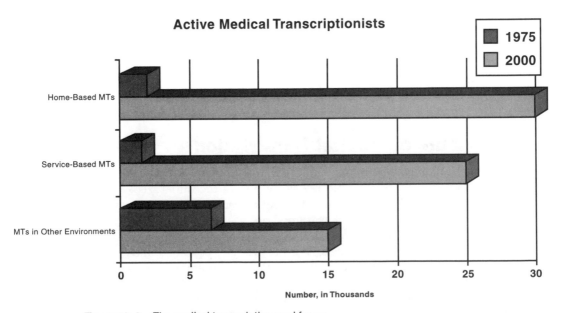

Figure 19–3   The medical transcription workforce

transcription training programs offered in major urban areas at institutions such as trade and technical schools, adult public education centers, city and community colleges, correspondence courses, and private tutorial settings. To further legitimize its standing as a career separate from clerical and medical assistant positions, the U. S. Department of Labor has designated separate codes (**SICs,** or standard industry codes) and titles for medical transcription as an occupation.

Over the years, MTs have made significant strides in education, workplace opportunities, and income, and if current U. S. Department of Labor projections hold true, medical transcription will be one of the fastest-growing occupations in the twenty-first century.

Summary of Concepts

- The pros and cons of each medical transcription work environment are important in evaluating the best setting in which a new MT should pursue his or her career.
- Important factors in selecting a work environment include the hours worked, the work schedule, flexibility, the pay basis, the benefits offered, and the experience required.
- A temporary employment agency is a potential work environment for MTs.
- There are several advantages and disadvantages for new MTs pursuing a career in hospitals, specialty medical offices, and clinics/multispecialty medical offices, with medical transcription services and temporary agencies, and at home.
- The three health-care markets —urban, suburban, and rural—can influence the pay medical transcriptionists can expect to earn in the area in which they live and/or work.
- For each health-care market, there usually are a certain number of trauma care centers that provide emergency medical services for the population contained within that market. These trauma care centers are able to provide emergency medical services that decrease with the level of service, with Level 1 providing the highest level of service and Level 5 providing only minimal service.
- The pay a medical transcriptionist receives increases with market size—the larger the market, the greater the pay.
- Over the years, MTs have made significant strides in education, workplace opportunities, and income, and the outlook for MTs is promising.

Chapter 20

Marketing Your Medical Transcription Talents

Overview: After choosing a work environment, the medical transcriptionist must then decide how to obtain that all-important first job in medical transcription. What tools are needed for the first interview? How does the employment process proceed? What if you decide to become an independent medical transcriptionist instead of a medical transcription employee? This chapter will answer these questions and more as you pursue marketing your newly acquired medical transcription talents.

Key Words

addenda

additional skills activities, awards,
    accomplishments or qualifications

advertising

business cards

business plan

business purpose statement

chain of command

character

character reference

classified ads

client requirements

cold calling

commitment to detail

competition

cover letter

DOE

educational experience

educational qualifications

employment application

EOE

financial prospectus

flyers

font

font attributes

home-based MT

human resources department

Internet

interview

interviewer

letters of recommendation

mailers

new client checklist

personal communications

Personal Data Sheet

personnel office

placement office

potential clients

potential employer

pre-employment requisites

rate sheet

references

resume

resume packet

resume title

salary requirements

self-employment potential

service requirements

target market

vocational qualifications

want ads

work experience

work objective

work-related reference

20–A The Resume Packet

Once the medical transcriptionist begins looking for his or her first medical transcription position, he or she will need to possess certain **pre-employment requisites** (essentials needed to obtain a job). Some requisites will be things you sent to a prospective employer or brought to your first interview at your potential place of employment. Other requisites are intangible and constitute part of your "collective intelligence," as mentioned in Chapter 1.

One of the most important requisites is a document that is considered one of the most helpful tools when a person is pursuing a new occupation—a resume.

The Resume

In its most basic form, a **resume** is a brief summary of a person's career and qualifications for the career she or he is pursuing. In its most effective form, a resume is a detailed sequential overview of an individual's career objectives, **educational qualifications** (schooling), **vocational qualifications** (past jobs), special skills, awards and accomplishments, and references, both character and professional. (See Figure 20–1.) Sometimes a resume is referred to as a **Personal Data Sheet.**

As detailed in Chapter 7, the curriculum vitae (CV) is a more comprehensive resume that includes items such as publications, association memberships, continuing education, and all experience pertinent to one's career. Individuals who have many qualifications sometimes combine sections normally included in a CV with those typically included in a resume to form a more comprehensive review.

Following are the items that should be included when sending a resume to a prospective employer. Together, these items constitute the **resume packet.** Include in your resume packet, in the following order, the cover letter, resume, references, and **addenda** (other correspondence including salary requirement statements, list of publications, sample work, etc.), if necessary. Use the following notes as guidelines when preparing your resume packet.

Cassandra Metropoulos
10015 East Park Avenue
Marysville, NY 01001-3604
Phones: 212-555-1234 (voice)
212-555-9876 (fax) / 212-555-0000 (modem)

OBJECTIVE: To procure employment as a medical transcriptionist in a medical office/clinic setting

EDUCATION: Branson Community College - Branson, New York
September XXXX to present
Associate of Science (A.S.) degree in Medical Transcription (to be conferred 6/10/XX)

Hamlet High School - New York, New York
September XXXX to June XXXX
High School (H.S.) diploma, with honors

WORK EXPERIENCE: Externship (non-compensated position)
Medical Offices of John Baker, M.D., Gastroenterologist
Branson, New York
October XXXX to April XXXX
Supervisor: Marta Svensen, Medical Office Administrator
Duties: Medical transcription, medical administrative assisting

Sal's Pizza World
Mountainberg, New York
July XXXX to December XXXX
Supervisor: Sal Monera, Owner
Duties: Preparing and baking various home-style cooked dishes including pizza, pasta and salads

OTHER SKILLS AND QUALIFICATIONS: Typing speed of 85 words per minute (w.p.m.)
Have access to own word processing equipment including Pentium personal computer, fax/modem and inkjet printer

AWARDS: Class salutatorian, Hamlet High School, June XXXX
Member, National Honor Society

REFERENCES: Marta Svensen, Medical Office Administrator, 212-555-5050
Vicki Kwansa, Paramedic, 212-555-8642

Figure 20–1   A resume

General Resume Guidelines

1. A resume should never contain the word "resume" as a title or other part of the resume. The **resume title** is usually the individual's name, address and phone number(s).

2. Single space the resume with at least one-half inch margins on the left, right, top and bottom sides. Usually, one-inch margins are preferred.

3. A resume should be keyed, word processed, typeset, and/or printed using a type size (**font**) that is readable and simple. Never use script and try to use only simple **font attributes** (italicization, underlining, all capitalization and bold print) when necessary.

4. Do not include abbreviations on a resume (except with dates and postal state and country codes) or contractions. Always spell out degree names such as Associate of Science degree in Mathematics, Bachelor of Arts degree in Mass Communications, and Master of Science degree in Computer Science, but you may also use a combination of spelling out the words followed by parenthetical abbreviations of the degree [e.g., "Master of Social Work degree (M.S.W.)", "Medical Doctor degree (M.D.)"].

5. List your most current qualifications first, in descending chronological order (i.e., college education would be listed before high school education; most current job would be listed before past jobs).

6. Use nine-digit U.S. postal codes on your resume, if you know them.

7. Use your full name on a resume (it is not necessary to include middle names, maiden names, etc., if you typically do not use them).

8. Print your resume on high-quality paper such as bond, laser quality, linen or other similar professional-looking paper. You may use colored paper, but make sure it is not overwhelming or distracting and that the print is easy to read. Use the same paper for your cover letter and resume, and try to use a matching envelope.

9. Everything on your resume should be honest and valid, however, always emphasize your strengths and assets, and deemphasize or omit your weaknesses. If you do not feel your resume demonstrates that you have the necessary experience for the job you are seeking, include a full explanation in your cover letter about why you feel you would be a good candidate for the position.

10. Make sure your resume is neat, clean and professional looking. Keep in mind that the resume represents you. Also, never use staples, paper clips, tape or any other type of fastener on your resume. Leave each page of your resume packet detached but in order. Send the resume packet in a legal-sized envelope measuring at least 9" × 11½". Folding the resume is not advised unless the employer requests that the resume be sent in a standard business-sized envelope (a #10 envelope measuring 9½" × 4⅛") where folding into thirds would be necessary.

Resume Sections

1. *Resume title* (your name, address and phone number). (Again, at no time should any portion of your resume contain the word "resume.") In the **resume title** section, include your full name, address including apartment

number, box number or suite, city, state and postal (zip) code, and all phone numbers where you can be reached, including voice telephone, fax phone number, and modem connection number, if you have these. Do not include on your resume the times you can be reached; this may be explained in the cover letter. Also, do not include personal information that could be used in a discriminatory way against you, such as race, gender, marital status, number of children, health, birth date or birthplace (as well as other private personal information such as height, weight, and Social Security number) on your resume. These items were once commonly included on resumes but no longer fall within the realm of necessary resume material. You may supply some of this information if you are comfortable doing so, and if asked for, on an employment application.

2. *Work objective.* The **work objective,** often called "Career Objective" or simply "Objective," contains a statement regarding what type of job you are looking for and why you are qualified. It usually is styled in the following format: "OBJECTIVE: To obtain [or attain, procure, achieve, gain, etc.] a position in the field of medical transcription [or other career name(s)] where my talents and skills [or abilities, accomplishments, experience, enthusiasm for job, people-helping skills, etc.] can be well utilized [or used well]." Always include this section immediately after your name on the resume so the prospective employer will at once know who you are and what it is you are looking for.

3. *Educational experience.* In the **educational experience** section, include all secondary (high school level) and post-secondary (college level) schools and courses you have attended. If it has been more than five years since you graduated from high school, do not include secondary school information, unless specifically asked for on an application.

4. *Work experience.* In the **work experience** section, include all pertinent (related) work experience. If you do not have any pertinent work experience, include in this section nonrelated work experience, volunteer work, internships and externships, and so on. If your work experience is more significant than your educational experience, include this category before the educational experience section.

5. *Additional skills, activities, awards, accomplishments, or qualifications* for the position. Include in this section any **additional skills, activities, awards, accomplishments,** or **qualifications** to date. This includes all extracurricular (outside of school and work) activities in which you have excelled. Activities may be related to both education and/or work but are not specific educational or work experiences. List any awards or recognitions you may have received, any additional skills such as typing speed, production speed in words per minute or lines per hour, or any other abilities or accomplishments you feel may help you succeed in getting the job you seek. If your list of accomplishments and awards is lengthy and noteworthy, you may choose to include this section before the educational and work experience categories.

6. *References.* In this section, include at least two character and/or work-related references. A **character reference** is someone to whom questions

regarding one's **character** (specific traits including appearance, attitude or behavior, and methods of problem solving, reliability, promptness, etc.) can be addressed. A **work-related reference** is someone with whom you have previously worked. Although a work-related reference could be a former co-worker, he or she usually is a previous supervisor or manager, or someone who was once in a position to evaluate your work skills and abilities. All references should be persons who are familiar with you and, if asked, would give you a favorable recommendation letter. Assume that these references will be contacted. Always include a name, company, title (or relationship, if friend or relative), phone, and, if space allows, a current address. If you would include with your resume more than three references, list them on a separate sheet of paper.

The Cover Letter

The cover letter is another important part of the resume packet. A **cover letter** is a typed or word processed correspondence that introduces you to a prospective employer. It describes in sentence form your career or work objective, it further outlines your specific qualifications for the job, and it explains why you would be a good candidate for the job. It conveys when you are available to work and what type of work you are looking for (e.g., part time, full time, temporary, etc.). It also provides a summary of any additional experience you may have. Finally, it should include a sentence thanking the potential employer for her or his time and telling the employer how they can best contact you. As with the resume, never include the words "cover letter" in the actual cover letter.

Some employers request that a cover letter be included with the resume; others want just the resume. Include a cover letter unless otherwise instructed. When mailing a resume packet, indicate that a resume is enclosed. When faxing a resume packet, indicate that a resume is attached. (See Figure 20–2.)

Addenda

The following additional documents may accompany your resume and cover letter. Enclose them if instructed to do so or if you feel they will aid you in gaining employment. Keep in mind that additional information can be distracting to the potential employer; you want your resume packet to be concise and focused on your qualifications as they relate to procuring the position listed in your objective.

Additional References   In addition to the character and work-related references noted on your resume, you may want to enclose an additional reference sheet. On this sheet you may wish to list additional references, additional information about previously noted references, or different categories of references (such as "Colleague References" or "Instructor References"). Again, do not enclose this sheet if you have three or fewer references.

Salary Requirements   Include a statement of your **salary requirements** only if instructed to do so. Most salary (pay) issues are discussed at the initial interview with an employer, and even in these cases you would be well advised to say that you are "flexible" or "open" when discussing your salary requirements, unless you are an expert in the field and obviously command a high salary. Many

Cassandra Metropoulos
10015 East Park Avenue
Marysville, NY 01001-3604

May 23, XXXX

Angelica Barrelos, A.R.T., R.R.A.
Medical Records Director
Columbia Hospital
5000 Main Street
White Plains, NY 01234

Fax #: 212-555-8989

Dear Ms. Barrelos:

I am corresponding in response to your advertisement for a medical transcriptionist in the May 16 edition of the *New York Times*. I am excited about the potential of working with a company such as yours. Attached please find my resume and salary requirement statement, as requested in your ad.

When you peruse my resume, you will find that I am new to the field of medical transcription. I am currently finishing my medical transcription studies at Branson Community College (BCC) in Branson, New York. I am scheduled to graduate in early June and will receive an Associate of Science degree. I have gained a great deal of experience transcribing authentic medical dictation at BCC including a six-month externship at the office of Dr. John Baker, a gastroenterologist in Branson. I was also quite active in my local chapter of AAMT while a student at BCC.

During my BCC externship at Dr. Baker's office I performed a variety of gastroenterology-related transcription including transcribing chart notes, medical correspondence, and gastrointestinal procedure notes such as barium swallows, upper GI procedures, and esophagogastroduodenoscopies. I also performed a variety of medical administrative assisting duties such as scheduling, telephone answering, completing insurance forms, and records filing while serving my externship at Dr. Baker's office.

If you agree that my educational experience, eagerness to learn, and enthusiasm for the job complement your needs for the position of medical transcriptionist at Columbia Hospital, please contact me at 212-555-1234 at your convenience.

Sincerely,

Cassandra Metropoulos

Cassandra Metropoulos

Attachments

Figure 20–2   A cover letter

positions include the abbreviation **DOE** (Depending On Experience). If you are new to the field, you will not have a tremendous amount of experience and should be realistic and flexible in your salary expectations.

However, if a potential employer requests that you state your salary requirements, type a brief letter with a statement such as, "My salary requirements are negotiable," contained within the letter. If there indeed is a minimum amount you need, do indicate that this is the case within the letter. You might say something such as, "Within the scope of my current financial situation, I would prefer to earn at least $__ per hour, although I am certainly flexible on this issue." Do not overemphasize the reason or explain in great detail why you are making such a statement. Again, include salary requirement statements in your resume packet only if specifically requested.

Letters of Recommendation   **Letters of recommendation** are certainly helpful companions to your resume. (See Figure 20–3.) Again, only include them if you feel they are necessary to convey your qualifications to a potential employer or if they are specifically requested. You should advise character, work-related, educational and other references to make their letters short and concise. They should be addressed, "To Whom It May Concern." They can be addressed in care of your address or the address can be left blank. The salutation should read, "Dear Madam or Sir:" or something similar. Do not enclose more than three letters of recommendation unless they are specifically requested.

Other Addenda   Other addenda can include samples of previous work (e.g., sample transcription for a medical transcriptionist position, clippings for a position as a writer, examples of edited copy for an editor position), required forms, copies of certificates, college transcripts, and so on. Again, only include these other addenda if specifically requested by the potential employer or if you feel they would increase your chances of being selected by an employer.

20–B The Employment Process

The employment process is a five-step one. Each rung of the ladder to employment must be climbed to fulfill your objective of becoming employed. First you must find out about job openings in your field. Next, you must apply and/or send a resume packet to the prospective employer. If you are selected as a potential candidate for employment, you will then be scheduled for an interview with a representative from the potential employer's hiring department (also called the **personnel office** or the **human resources department** in larger facilities). If you are selected to proceed further in the employment process, you will likely be scheduled for a second (and sometimes third) interview, usually with a supervisor, manager, physician or other facility staff member who will be directly supervising you or working with you if you acquire the position. If you pass this final scrutinization, you will likely be asked to join the facility. Anyone who has patience, perseverance, a commitment to succeed, and a good attitude can and will achieve this goal.

John Baker, M.D., F.A.C.S.

GASTROENTEROLOGY • GASTROESOPHAGEAL SURGERY

300 Park Avenue • Suite 2050 • Branson, New York 01111

(212) 555-1111

Staff:

Brandy Smith, P.A.-C
Physician's Assistant

Madeline Waters, C.R.T.
Radiology Technician

Marta Svensen
Administrator

May 10, XXXX

To Whom It May Concern
c/o Cassandra Metropoulos
10015 East Park Avenue
Marysville, NY 01001-3604

Dear Madam or Sir:

It is with great pride that I offer my highest recommendation for Ms. Cassandra Metropoulos. She served her externship with our office from last October until April of this year.

Cassandra's skills in medical transcription are far more advanced than would be anticipated from her brief education in the field. She demonstrates patience, flexibility and understanding when working with others, and she reacts well to instruction and criticism. Cassandra is a quick learner and when presented with multiple tasks she carries each of them out in a logical and efficient manner. She consistently displays positive interaction with both patients and co-workers. She always respects patient and physician confidentiality. Working with Cassandra is truly a pleasure.

If you have any questions or would like to discuss her medical transcription qualifications in greater detail, please contact me.

Sincerely,

Marta Svensen

Marta Svensen
Office Administrator

MS:mtl

Figure 20–3　A letter of recommendation

Step 1: Discover Employment Opportunities

The first step to becoming employed as a medical transcriptionist (or any occupation) is to find out who is offering employment. The most common way of discovering employment opportunities is the "Help Wanted" portion of the classified section of your local newspaper. The **classified ads** provide a categorical listing of advertisements such as available employment positions, real estate, items for sale, and so on. Sunday newspapers usually provide the largest volume of classified ads and also the greatest assortment of employment opportunity advertisements or "**want ads**." (See Figure 20–4 for a sample "want ad.")

When you are scanning the help wanted ads, first look for positions listed under the section entitled "Health Care" or "Health Related," if there is one; if there is not such a section, look alphabetically under the letter "M" for "medical transcription." Sometimes medical transcription ads are listed under "T" for "transcription" in the health-care section. Also look for positions listed under the following categories: "medical records," "medical administrative," "medical assisting—front office," and "secretary—medical." If no matching ads are found, look under the more general employment categories to see whether anything meets the description of a medical transcription position being offered. Also look

MEDICAL TRANSCRIPTIONIST

Due to recent expansion in our medical records department, Children's Hospital of Philadelphia is currently seeking a trained medical transcriptionist. Duties will include transcription of "basic four" reports on the Wang word processing system. Familiarity with Lanier remote digital dictation equipment is highly recommended. Position is for full-time, day shift (8:00 to 4:30 p.m.), including occasional weekend and swing shift rotations. At least one year medical transcription experience or training at an accredited post-secondary institution is required for this position. Medical, dental, life and a 401(k), as well as continuing education assistance, is offered as part of this employment package. Fax your resume today to: Human Resources, Children's Hospital of Philadelphia, at 555-1221. Salary DOE. EOE.

MEDICAL TRANSCRIPTION

Two radiology transcription positions available. One P/T flexible, one F/T days. At least 2 yrs. exp in hospital radiology transcription pref'd. Salary is based on production. Fill out an application at our office Mon.-Wed. Eastern Radiology, 3333 Magnolia Ct. S.E., Philadelphia, 555-3333. No phone calls please.

Figure 20–4   Sample employment opportunity advertisements

at display (large, usually boxed or lined ads, that list more than one position) ads for medical transcription positions.

Although Sunday papers usually have the most comprehensive listing of help wanted ads, also check the daily classified ads to learn about other opportunities. (Sometimes if an employer lists a position during the week it means that they are eager to fill the position or that they are not receiving enough qualified applicants.)

In addition to the want ads, you may discover employment opportunities through the following: a hospital personnel office or an open-jobs listing posted elsewhere in a hospital or other large medical facility; public or private employment agencies (be sure to find out if there are any fees associated with the services of an employment agency; if there are, find out who is responsible for paying those fees, the employee or the employer), temporary employment agencies (see Chapter 19); community bulletin boards (for example, in grocery stores) or computer bulletin boards; computer on-line services and the **Internet** (the World Wide Web); special employment literature (such as a "Job Paper" or other similar publication); the **placement office** of a college, trade school, or other educational facility (see if you are eligible to receive this type of job placement service, especially at a school you once attended), health-care magazines, medical journals and other medical periodicals (such as the ones published by a local or regional medical society); and finally through "word of mouth" (i.e., a friend or colleague hears about a possible job opening at a medical facility). You can also find out about jobs that are not yet advertised by visiting personnel offices, keeping apprised of new or expanding medical practices, and contacting medical facilities listed in the yellow pages of telephone directories (check under these and other listings: "clinics", "hospitals", "physicians", etc.). Always keep in mind that all employment opportunities should be open to all persons, regardless of sex, race, ethnic or cultural heritage, religion, creed, age or physical disability (many employers state "**EOE**" or "Equal Opportunity Employer" in their ads for employment).

Step 2: Begin the Application Process

Once you find one or more ads or other employment offerings you feel you may be qualified for, you must make contact with the prospective employer. Carefully follow the instructions in the ad or job listing. If you are instructed not to call but the ad lists a phone number, do not call. If you are instructed to fax a copy of your resume, do so. If you do not own a fax machine, most larger grocery stores, business supply stores or other office settings will usually let you use their fax machines for a nominal fee. If you are instructed to apply in person, find out the hours of the facility and plan to visit the correct location (within the times and on the dates specified, if indicated). If you are instructed to submit a resume, do so but do not visit the location in addition to submitting your resume without prior authorization. (See the previous Section 20–A for tips on submitting a resume.) Duplication of applications can occur if you apply for a position in more than one manner.

If you are asked to visit the prospective place of employment to fill out an **employment application** (official form on which you apply for a position with a company), bring your resume. If an application is sent to you, fill it out while consulting your resume.

You should always be consistent, accurate and thorough when completing the employment application. Guidelines for completing the employment application follow:

1. Read all instructions carefully. This is often stated on the application form; however, because many applicants are rushing through the process or are nervous, they may disregard this important advice. Remember, relax and take your time. Completing the application accurately and neatly is a very important part of the employment process, and if you fail to do so you may have to start all over again with a different employer.

2. Read the entire form, unless instructed not to do so. Before answering any questions or filling in any blank spaces, make sure you thoroughly understand what information the employer is looking for. Be on the lookout for special instructions such as "Last name first" or "Dates in numbers with dashes."

3. Fill out the form in its entirety. Provide accurate and well-thought-out answers to all questions asked. If for some reason you cannot provide a response when asked to do so, or if the question does not apply to you, do not leave the area blank. Write "N/A" (meaning "not appropriate") or "none" in the space allotted for your response. Also, if questions are asked and the response would be the same as in prior responses, you may write "same as above," making sure it is clear what the response is intended to indicate.

4. If asked, provide salary requirements, or the amount of pay you are expecting. You may respond to this question by answering "negotiable", or "open" or you may specify a salary range (such as 7 to 8 cents per line). Avoid providing an inflexible salary figure; there usually is room for advancement and pay raises further down the road, once you secure the position.

5. Attach a copy of your resume. Again, do not physically attach the resume with a fastener, but place a copy of the resume underneath the application.

6. Carefully double check your answers. Make sure each answer is correct and complete and corresponds to the information given in your resume. Then ask yourself these questions: Have I answered all questions and not left any blank spaces or unfinished answers? Have I confined my answers to the spaces allocated? Have I avoided any extraneous marks? Have I made the best possible representation of myself on this application? If the answer to each of these questions is yes, you have properly completed the application.

Sometimes testing and an initial interview also are done at the time the application is completed. Be prepared for this. The testing might include, but not be limited to, the following items: a typing test, to determine your typing speed and accuracy level; a word processing knowledge test, to determine your dexterity and skill with word processing software you may have indicated you are familiar with; a medical terminology test, to evaluate your knowledge of medical terms and their correct spellings; a medical transcription mechanics test, to evaluate your knowledge of formatting, such as word usage, capitalization, abbreviations, and so on; and one or more tests, such as grammar, to evaluate your general command of the English language. You will score higher on these types of tests if you keep the following points in mind:

1. *Prepare yourself for the test beforehand.* Administer self-tests, including typing speed and word processing knowledge tests. Give yourself oral and written terminology tests. Review study materials for things such as medical transcription mechanics, formats and grammar.
2. *Relax and take your time.* Try not to be anxious or nervous. Use your time wisely and do not rush through a test. Testing should reflect your average abilities and skills. Keep in mind that this is not the only portion of the application process that counts. Remember, if you put your best foot forward and have a good attitude you will succeed.
3. *Keep your eyes open for hints within a test.* You may find that answers to a section of a test can be found in previous questions.

Step 3: Pass the First Interview

As mentioned previously, once your application and/or resume has been reviewed, you are often scheduled for an **interview** with the person who hires new employees. This question-and-answer session, with you providing the majority of the answers to questions the **interviewer** presents to you, may be done as soon as you complete your application or may be scheduled for a later date.

You also may be told that you will be notified if you are selected for an interview. If you do not hear from a **potential employer** (someone who may hire you), do not call their office. Instead, write a short note indicating your continued interest in the position, but try not to make repeated attempts to contact the potential employer or to become an annoyance. It usually is best to let the potential employer contact you. To ensure that you do not miss that important call, you should have access to a telephone answering machine, a voice mail system, or another reliable way to receive messages. If you do not hear any further information from a potential employer within a reasonable period of time (usually four weeks) after your application or resume has been submitted, assume that the position has been filled. However, do not take this personally; it may just mean this was not the right job for you and that another, possibly a better job opportunity, will become available.

If you are scheduled for a first interview, or if the interview is given simultaneously with submission of your application, be prepared. Know every detail of your resume. Make sure you can fulfill all of the necessary job requirements. Be prepared to answer questions such as why you left a previous position, what goals you may have in this new position, and why you are seeking this particular position. Be familiar with the employer, the exact duties of the position, and the work schedule. If you have any questions, ask them. Know beforehand the expected salary and benefits for similar positions with your level of education and experience so you will be prepared if these issues are discussed. You might consider staging a "mock" interview, where a friend or relative acts as the interviewer and poses sample questions to you.

At the first interview, keep the following points in mind:

1. Dress and groom yourself properly, in a businesslike manner. Remember, your first impression is a lasting one, which carries a lot of weight when deciding whether or not you are the right person for the job. Dress in business attire—suit and tie if male, a skirt, dress, or pantsuit if female. Make sure your shoes

are clean and your clothing is fresh and pressed. Observe proper hygiene and do not use excessive amounts of scented soaps, colognes or perfumes; the odors may be offensive to your potential employer and to others.

2. Maintain a cheerful, positive attitude throughout the interview. Bring a resume or other items with you so you do not appear nervous, anxious or fidgety. Always smile and try to appear relaxed. If your voice cracks or fades, simply ask for a glass of water.

3. Allow the interviewer to direct the interview; simply respond to questions in the most organized, complete and thoughtful manner possible. Provide more than simple "yes" or "no" responses to questions, but be as brief as possible while conveying exactly what you would like to say.

4. Smile and maintain eye contact with the interviewer. Do not stare, but look the interviewer in the eye from time to time, especially when you are responding to questions. Use your normal style when speaking, but keep nodding and overt facial expressions to a minimum.

5. Ask the interviewer any questions you may have regarding the position when appropriate, but be concise and to the point. You may want to write down possible questions to pose to the employer prior to going to the interview. Make sure the questions do not deal exclusively with issues the employer will discuss, such as salary, time off, and so on. Categorize your questions in descending order of importance to ensure that your highest-priority questions are answered first.

6. Finally, look for clues from the interviewer regarding where the conversation is going. Some interviews are short, others are long. Usually the interviewer controls the length of the interview. Do not appear as though you are ready to leave before the interviewer indicates that the interview is finished. When the interviewer appears to be concluding the interview, make sure to thank her or him for taking the time to speak to you. If you have not previously given a copy of your resume to the interviewer, be prepared to give him or her a copy at this time. Tell the interviewer that you look forward to speaking with her or him again and to the possibility of working with the potential employer.

Step 4: Sail through the Second (or Third) Interview

Once the initial interviewer has reviewed your responses and your application and/or resume, you may be asked back for a second or third interview. These subsequent interviews will likely be with a more immediate supervisor or manager, or someone who has decision-making power in terms of your possible employment, such as a physician or other medical staff member. By this time, you are probably a very good candidate for the position. You also will likely be somewhat more familiar with the facility, its personnel and procedures and the employer's expectations. You will probably be more relaxed at subsequent interviews than you were during the first one. However, be sure to keep the same basic guidelines in mind whenever you are interviewing with a potential employer: 1) dress and groom yourself properly, in a businesslike manner; 2) maintain a cheerful, positive attitude throughout the interview; 3) allow the interviewer to direct the interview; 4) smile and maintain eye contact with the interviewer; 5) ask any questions you may have, but be concise and to the point; and 6) look for clues from the interviewer regarding where the conversation is going. Even if the interviewer is a physician or other highly trained and experienced medical practitioner, try not to feel intimidated or shy. Remember, the interviewer is a person, just like yourself, and would likely react similarly if he or she were in your shoes.

After a final interview, all of your qualifications and interview responses will be carefully evaluated. If you are qualified for the position, have given logical, appropriate, and truthful answers, and the employer feels you have the qualities necessary for successful employment with their facility, you no doubt will achieve employment.

Step 5: Get the Job

Once you have successfully passed Step 4, you most likely will be hired. Congratulations on your new career! Gaining employment, however, is not your final goal. You still have many things to learn about your new workplace and career. Always strive for improvement in yourself and in your career.

The following guidelines will help you succeed in your new endeavor:

1. Observe routines, take notes and ask questions once you are on the job.
2. Always keep the lines of communication open.
3. Maintain a good relationship with your supervisor, and make sure to always follow the proper **chain of command** (correct procedure for flow of communication between you, your supervisors and their supervisors—those higher in the office hierarchy).
4. Your employer will no doubt realize that you are new to the job and may make mistakes; however, learn from your mistakes instead of repeating them.
5. Address problems immediately instead of letting them accumulate.
6. Keep **personal communications** (phone calls, visits, conversations with co-workers, etc.) to a minimum.
7. Continue your education. Seek out courses, seminars and other training opportunities that will help you advance in your career.
8. Become active in your profession. Join professional organizations (such as AAMT), attend company functions, and seek out colleagues to share those experiences.

20–C On Your Own: The Independent Medical Transcriptionist

As previously stated, it usually is more beneficial for a medical transcriptionist who is new to the profession to work outside of the home or as a subcontractor for a period of at least six months before becoming an independent contractor. Once you have enough experience, however, you may be interested in pursuing this career option. Becoming a **home-based MT** provides the person who is motivated and committed an opportunity to control her or his own schedule, work load, and paycheck. The paycheck can be quite substantial (see Chapter 19, Figure 19–1) for someone who is fast, makes a significant time commitment, and produces consistent error-free, high-quality work.

Would becoming a home-based independent medical transcriptionist be the best career move for you? If you want to succeed, consider reviewing the following necessary steps prior to deciding whether or not this is the right course of action for you.

Step 1: Determine your self-employment potential

Some medical transcriptionists make the decision to work independently well before they know what lies ahead. Some are new to the career and have inadequate experience to establish themselves as home-based MTs. Others make the move to the MT career from another home-based occupation, without being fully aware of exactly what the business of medical transcription entails. Then there are experienced MTs who have never before worked at home and have difficulty adjusting to the independent MT lifestyle. These pitfalls do not have to be your destiny. However, you must be prepare yourself. Working at home on your own schedule literally whenever and however you choose takes a lot of hard work, dedication and ability. In addition to drive, determination and business savvy, running any business successfully also requires a healthy amount of preparation. Before you seriously consider working as a home-based medical transcriptionist, you may want to ask yourself the following questions to help determine your **self-employment potential** as a home-based MT.

1. *Am I qualified to become a home-based MT?* A qualified home-based MT candidate will have had formal education in medical terminology and transcription and the equivalent of at least six months' experience transcribing medical reports, correspondence, office charting and other documents. The successful home-based MT candidate will also have had experience transcribing dictation that involves a variety of terminology, formats, and dictator pronunciations and dialects. This experience can be gained through working in a medical environment (one of the previously discussed medical transcription environments), in an externship or internship as an MT, or working at home as an MT under the direction of a more experienced medical transcriptionist.

2. *If I want to work in my own community, am I located in the correct market?* A market conducive to home-based medical transcription for an experienced MT would be an urban or a suburban market with a large and diverse base of **potential clients** (entities for whom you may perform a service in the future). If your community is a rural market and/or you have less than the recommended amount of experience, you may find it necessary to possess exemplary marketing skills (see later discussion) and have the necessary equipment, experience and desire to work as a subcontractor remote transcriptionist for a bigger MT service in a larger market.

3. *Am I detail- and quality-oriented and motivated to act without a deadline? Am I a self-starter?* Home-based independent medical transcription requires a 100 percent **commitment to detail** (you must be good at editing, proofreading, and researching problems) and quality (you should make fewer than two errors per page with normal transcription of complex dictation). A home-based MT also must be able to start and complete a project not only within the time limitations of turnaround but also within the outer boundaries of time and work commitments to self, friends and family. In other words, you must be willing and able to start projects hours before facing an impending deadline.

4. *Am I disciplined enough to pass up a night on the town for a night of must-finish transcription?* Any home-based business demands much more attention than an identical career working under the direction of another. This is especially true in the case of medical transcription. You will often (if not always) find yourself working nights, weekends, and holidays when others around you are celebrating and enjoying themselves. There may be many distractions while you work, such as the doorbell or telephone ringing, faxes being received, family members needing your assistance, and so on. You may be dismayed when those who dictate take the day off or do not work on a holiday, because that will mean no or little pay for you that day. You will hear about the plans of others and long to get away yourself, but know you cannot because you have a deadline. With the tremendous time commitment to your career, you will make a good income but will sacrifice much of your time to transcription.

5. *Can I work in the absence of others?* Some people are real "people people"; in other words, they like working and dealing with people in their daily occupational environment. Home-based medical transcription entails working on your own with very few distractions and no co-workers. You will not have much interaction with others, especially patients, doctors and other medical personnel. Working on your own probably means missing out on such things as office parties and holiday bonuses, office chitchat, and company picnics. You may never even the chance to meet some of the office staff you work with daily over the phone.

6. *Do I have a good business sense?* Home-based medical transcription requires a working knowledge of marketing, bookkeeping, public relations and networking. The successful home-based MT will know how to go about getting new clients and keeping the ones they have, how to keep good financial and other business-oriented records, how to advertise, how to keep clients happy and put on the best face possible in times of adversity, and how to communicate, interact and intermingle with colleagues you can help and who can be of valuable assistance to you. Operating a home-based business requires knowing the advantages and disadvantages of the legal aspects of setting up your business as a sole proprietorship, a partnership or a corporation. Financial and tax issues arise from time to time, and good business owners will know when they can handle the matter on their own and when they need to consult with other experts. Business owners must be risk takers to some degree, but they also must able to realize when the potential cost of any planned venture does not justify the possible loss associated with that risk.

If you answered yes to all of the previous questions, you are probably ready to start planning a future as a home-based medical transcriptionist. If you answered negatively to one or more of the questions, you might want to gain some further experience and detect and implement any changes necessary to make a home-based MT career work for you.

Step 2: Formulate a Business Plan

So you are on your way to becoming an independent home-based medical transcriptionist. You will not get very far, however, without first developing a plan of action and implementation for your home-based career, or a **business plan.** The business plan is both a conceptual plan and a tangible, written plan of action. In it, you must structure how you will set up your business, your goals, financial aspects concerning the business, materials you will need before beginning, and other things necessary to operate a business. Start with a simple outline of your business plan. Begin to slowly develop the plan until you have worked out even the most minute details. Then make it your goal to implement the plan. Some things you may want to include in your business plan include:

1. *Define your business purpose, mission, or goal.* This purpose statement clarifies why you want to go into business for yourself. The **business purpose statement** could be as simple as, "The purpose of this home-based independent medical transcription service will be to provide quality transcription at a reasonable cost in the most timely, orderly, and accurate fashion as possible." It could also be quite detailed, elaborating upon every aspect of your business that will set it apart from your competition.

2. *Define your target market and your competition.* Who will your potential clients be? Will your **target market** include physicians' offices or hospitals, medical offices, or local trauma centers? Who else in the transcription business is trying to get new accounts? Will your **competition** consist of other similarly trained and skilled independent home-based MTs, or large medical transcription services with annual revenues in the millions of dollars? Once you know who you will be competing against for new clients, you will have a better idea about how to proceed with challenging that competition.

3. *State your qualifications to begin a home-based business.* You will probably want to have on hand a current resume, a personal data sheet that includes more information than a resume (such as birth date, Social Security number, family information, personal and professional goals, interests and hobbies, etc.), a financial net worth sheet, and current references and letters of recommendation. You will no doubt need to refer to or present each of these at some point in presenting your business plan to others who can be of assistance to you. You will also need to document that your potential home-based business will have adequate space, amenities, and supplies to operate as a business out of your home.

4. *Formulate a financial prospectus.* The **financial prospectus** should include projections of monthly revenue and expenses for a two-year period, a personal or existing business (if you already have one in place) balance sheet, an estimation of start-up and operating costs and working capital, potential funding sources, and other financial worksheets.

5. *Analyze the potential strengths and risks involved with your business venture.* List the strengths, pinpoint the weaknesses, and discuss any risks that might be involved with starting your business (such as not being able to quickly acquire accounts, difficulty collecting debts, etc.). You should also cover aspects such as how much you intend to charge for your services (your **rate sheet**), making sure your cost is in line with the competition, how you plan to bill and collect, how you will retain clients, and other risk-related issues.

Step 3: Market Potential Clients

Your biggest and first challenge will be landing that important first client. To do so, you must market (sell) your skills as a medical transcriptionist to that client.

You must convince the potential client that you are not only skilled and experienced, but that there is something unique about you that makes you a better choice than your competition.

How and where do you go about getting the new client? There are several possible methods; choose one or a combination of those that best suit your individual marketing style.

Cold Calling This is probably the easiest and yet most challenging method of marketing. **Cold calling** involves simply picking up a telephone directory, looking under listings such as physicians, clinics, and hospitals, and making calls, lots of calls, trying to sell your medical transcription service. Other sources for obtaining names of potential clients include local chambers of commerce, medical societies, health-care magazine classifieds, newspaper ads, mailing label services, the Internet, colleagues, and your educational facility's placement service.

Prepare for cold calling by making a short list (20 or so names), a small goal (perhaps one or two "possibilities," or clients who may be interested now or at some point in the future), and a time frame (e.g., four hours). You should attempt to consistently make the same number of phone calls each day for a one- or two-week period of time. You will need a phone, a phone number, and a mailing address (some MTs choose to maintain a mailing address that is separate from their home addresses for security reasons and privacy).

It is helpful to prepare and practice a script when you begin making cold calls. The script might go something like this: "Hello. I'm Sarah Smith and I'm an independent medical transcriptionist (my company's name is XYZ Medical Transcription Service). Has your office ever sent its medical transcription to an outside service?" If the response is yes, you would continue, "Great! If you wouldn't mind, I'd like to tell you a little bit about myself and what I do, and if you would be interested, I'd like to send you some information about my medical transcription service so you can have it on file if you find you may have the need for a small, client-centered medical transcription service."

Whether or not the client is interested in your services, you have given the office your name, your company name, and you probably have told them a little bit about what you do and why they might choose your service over the competition. If the client is interested, make a note and follow up by sending a small information packet that includes a brief outline of your business purpose and goals, as well as a resume, business cards, flyers, and whatever other marketing tools you may have. If the client is not interested, simply make a note to that effect and keep the name on file for future reference. Remember, cold calling is 95 percent rejection, but the 5 percent overall who are at least willing to receive information about your business will be worth the effort.

Mailers **Mailers,** or the mailing of **flyers** (short printed or typeset one-page brochures), are similar to cold calling but without the one-on-one interaction. Simply create a one-sheet brochure, which can be folded into two or three sections and mailed without an envelope. The mailer is an attention-grabbing marketing device that can outline any or all of the following items: your business purpose and goals, what services you provide to clients, your skills and personal qualifications, your rates for service, and how you can be contacted. (See Figure 20–5.) You

Finally. A Medical Transcriptionist as professional as you are. . .

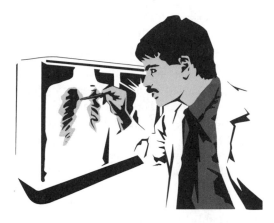

You're a medical professional and you like everything in your office done professionally. Things like your office notes. Your medical correspondence. Your office procedure notes. But you probably realize that it's difficult to get that professionalism in things like medical transcription. Well, professionalism has made a return.

My name is Chelsea Lake, and I am a professional home-based medical transcriptionist. I am the owner/transcriptionist of ABC Transcription Service of Marion, Texas.

As an experienced professional transcriptionist, I take things like accuracy, turnaround times and cost seriously. I have six months' experience in the medical specialties of psychiatry, otolaryngology and pathology medical transcription. I served an externship in medical transcription while attending classes at Susan B. Anthony VoTech right here in Washington County, Texas.

In my work as a medical transcriptionist I have encountered many types of dictation styles and dialects, and I am familiar with various medical

forms and formats. I am also a very quick learner.

I am eager to take on the challenge of satisfying your requirements of professionalism in medical transcription.

If you would be interested in discussing your medical transcription needs with me, now or at any point in the future, please just give me a call at (800) 555-5501 anytime.

ABC TRANSCRIPTION
1234 MAPLE LANE • MARION, TEXAS 77777
CHELSEA LAKE, OWNER/TRANSCRIPTIONIST
(800) 555-5501

Figure 20–5   A sample mailer/flyer

can mail this brochure at the least expensive postal rate to names you have selected from a telephone, medical, business or other type of directory. In addition to physicians and other health-care professionals, potential clients include depression and substance abuse facilities, rehabilitation centers, teaching universities, imaging (radiologic and other diagnostic procedure) centers, military bases, insurance agencies, legal offices and court reporting services, secretarial and word processing services, book and script authors, private investigators, and convention center services departments. Although this method of marketing is fairly inexpensive compared to others, do remember to include this cost on your expenses worksheet in your business plan.

Advertising   **Advertising** is usually the most expensive method of marketing. For a fee, from tens of dollars to thousands of dollars, you can put your name, company name, address, phone and sometimes a one-line (or more, if you can afford it) synopsis of what you do in most any type of publication. Your ad can be as simple as a telephone directory (yellow pages) listing, which usually costs a few hundred dollars for a small once-a-year listing, to a large, full-page ad in a hospital organization publication, such as the American Hospital Association's annual conference journal. You can purchase booths at medical conferences and seminars and can even host an event at these functions.

However, most home-based independent MTs simply do not have this kind of budget. Perhaps you could do something more practical as a newcomer to the home-based industry, such as placing a small one- or two-line ad in a local telephone directory of hospitals, physicians and clinics that is circulated only within that specific market. You could even have your own home page on the Internet with "hot keys" (sort of guidepost markers) that could direct potential clients to learn more about your service, the medical transcription business as a whole, medical transcription education, and so on. Remember to budget any advertising expenses into your financial prospectus.

Word of Mouth/Referrals   Word of mouth, networking, or simply getting referrals is probably the most economical and worry-free type of marketing for new clients. You will need a good supply of **business cards** (small calling cards containing at least your name, a company name, if you have one, an address, and your phone number—items such as artwork, a logo, etc., may be an unaffordable expense early on) and vigilant communication with colleagues, old school buddies, former instructors, medical office staff, and others. Take a small supply of business cards with you wherever you go and post them wherever you can (in grocery stores, churches, membership warehouse stores, groups and associations, bulletin boards, your doctor's office, etc.). Always ask permission to post your card. Also, try to enter raffles, drawings, and so on, where the merchant asks you to submit your business card (you may want to have an address other than your home address for this) so, if you happen to be a lucky winner or runner-up, you and your company might receive complimentary publicity.

In addition, try to attend all the medical transcription-related meetings, parties and other networking occasions you can, maintaining these contacts within the medical transcription community to provide further resources for you.

Step 4: Set Up the Account

Congratulations! You did it! You have landed your first client for whom you can perform medical transcription services. That client is now officially an "account." Whether the account is composed of overload dictation from a hospital, a physician's office dictation of chart notes and correspondence, or a personal injury law firm, you must do several things before beginning your work. You must totally understand the needs of your client to ensure that you are able to accommodate him or her. You must make sure the work will not overwhelm (or underwhelm) you. You must decide whether there will be enough consistency in the account to suffice as your only client, or whether you will need additional ones.

Make a **new client checklist** of the things you will need to know about the client and the things the client will need to know about you. Obviously you have discussed with them your rates. Will the client be doing holiday dictation? Are there after-hours business hours? Who do you contact when the office manager or contact is away? These types of questions, and any others you can think of, are crucial when setting up the account. Your checklist might include some of the items listed next. Whatever categories your checklist contains, make sure that when the checklist is completed you will have a clear understanding of your clients' needs and requests before you commit to taking on the account. Also be sure that the client understands exactly what services you will be providing and the cost for these services.

A sample checklist includes the following contents:

Client requirements:

1. What type of dictation (tape, remote, pickup and delivery, etc.)?
2. Turnaround time.
3. Volume of dictation (in minutes or other increments).
4. Frequency of dictation (e.g., every evening at 6:00 P.M. Monday through Friday, and Saturday at 12:00 noon).
5. Type of dictation (specialty terminology, formats, report forms, letterhead or stationery, sticky-back paper for chart notes, etc.).
6. Any special dictator needs (dialects or accents, specific pronunciations, abbreviations or terminology specific to the dictator, special degrees or affiliations of the dictator, instances in which to ask before editing, etc.).
7. Policy for returning completed transcription (printed out, on diskette, via modem, etc.).
8. Office holidays/policy on days when the dictator does not dictate.
9. Quality assurance/checking procedures and standards.

Service requirements (things you must know to properly service the account):

1. All client information, including contact name, full business name of client, pickup and mailing addresses, telephone numbers (including fax and after-hours numbers), billing attention line, bill submission method (bring bill to office, send through mail, etc.), and frequency of payment.
2. Type of accounting method client prefers (hourly wage, production by lines, words, bytes, etc.).

3. Individual office/facility policies (requesting sick time, reporting problems, office communication, backup measures [e.g., fill-ins for you, backup data storage, insurance, etc.]).
4. Collection policy (make invoice due within a certain number of days; if the client pays on time, perhaps offer a small discount).

Step 5: Maintain the Account

This is perhaps the most overlooked but one of the more important aspects of the home-based medical transcription service. After you have maintained an account for a few months or years, decide upon your next plan. Look back on your business plan in terms of goals you have made for yourself and your business to see if you have accomplished them; if so, what new goals can be set? And how do you make sure you retain your current accounts?

There are several ways to retain your account and keep your skills current.

1. *Ask for feedback.* Devise a "Customer Satisfaction Survey" and ask your clients for opinions of your work. Are they satisfied overall? Are their expectations being met in terms of turnaround, accuracy and overall quality? What could you do to improve your service? What could you do to help your clients improve their business (which will, in turn, make more business for you)?
2. *Refresh your skills.* Take a class or seminar in medical transcription or in a specific topic in the realm of health care or medicine. Ask your client (if appropriate) if you could do a one-week, in-house "pseudointernship" where you could observe the client going about day-to-day duties such as taking a patient's history or performing an operative procedure prior to dictating. Continue your education through extension classes, workshops, and computer-based learning programs.
3. *Stay up-to-date.* Constantly add new texts to your medical reference library. Join an on-line medical transcription discussion group. Keep abreast of the latest terminology and transcription techniques.

Always be on the lookout for new employment opportunities. Send holiday greetings, birthday cards, and "Just to keep in contact" notes to current and potential clients. Keep a supply of business cards handy. Always strive to be the best medical transcriptionist you can be. Never lose sight of the fact that your collective intelligence and experience is your greatest asset, and keep building upward. Good luck in your medical transcription career!

Summary of Concepts

- A resume is one of the most important pre-employment requisites and one of the most helpful tools for a person pursuing any new occupation.
- A resume is a brief summary of a person's work history and qualifications for the career she or he is pursuing, including career objectives, educational and vocational qualifications, special skills, awards and accomplishments, and references, both character and professional.

- The resume packet should include a cover letter, the resume, references, and addenda (other correspondence including salary requirement statements, a list of publications, sample work, etc.), if necessary.
- The employment process is a five-step one consisting of the following individual steps: 1) discover employment opportunities; 2) begin the employment application process; 3) pass the first interview; 4) sail through the second (or third) interview; and 5) get the job.
- Becoming a home-based MT provides an opportunity for someone who is experienced, motivated and committed to control her or his own schedule, workload, and paycheck.
- The process for assessing your potential for becoming a home-based independent medical transcriptionist includes the following individual steps: 1) determine your self-employment potential; 2) formulate a business plan; 3) market potential clients; 4) set up the account; and 5) maintain the account.
- Always be on the lookout for new work opportunities.

Appendices

Appendix A: Glossary of Common Medical Terms

abduct	(v.) to draw away from the body
acathisia, akathisia	(n.) a condition of motor restlessness; inability to remain inactive
accommodation	(n.) adjustment of the eye to distance
acute	(adj.) relating to a sudden and severe onset
adduct	(v.) to draw toward the body
adenoma	(n.) a glandular growth
adipose	(adj.) fatty; (n.) fat
adnexa	(n.) the accessory parts of a structure
aerobic	(adj.) pertaining to an absence of oxygen
afebrile	(adj.) without fever
alimentary	(adj.) pertaining to nutrition
allergen	(n.) a substance that induces hypersensitivity
ambulate	(v.) to walk or move about
amenorrhea	(n.) a condition of absence or cessation of menses
analgesic	(n.) a substance that relieves pain
anaphylaxis	(n.) severe hypersensitivity reaction to an allergen
anatomical	(adj.) pertaining to anatomy or body structure
anemia	(n.) a condition of having below the normal amount of erythrocytes
anesthetic	(adj.) producing loss of feeling or sensation or consciousness; (n.) an agent that induces decreased sensation or consciousness
aneurysm	(n.) abnormal localized widening of a blood vessel
angina	(n.) a condition producing severe pain and constriction of the heart that is a result of an insufficient blood supply to the heart
anomaly	(n.) something that deviates from normal
anorexia	(n.) loss of appetite; a condition marked by an inability to eat
antecubital	(adj.) in front of the elbow or in the fold of the arm
anterior	(adj.) pertaining to the front
anteverted	(adj.) tipped forward
antibiotic	(adj.) destructive of a living substance; (n.) a chemical microorganism substance that has the ability to destroy other microorganisms
antibody	(n.) an immunoglobulin molecule that interacts with or reacts to an antigen
antidote	(n.) a substance that counteracts a poison or a drug
anxiety	(n.) a feeling of unwarranted apprehension, uncertainty and/or fear, associated with physiological changes
Apgar score	a method of rating a newborn's physical condition at one minute and five minutes after birth, including appearance (color), pulse (heart rate), grimacing (stimulation response), activity (muscle tone), and respiratory rate
aphasia	(n.) inability to speak
apnea	(n.) a period of cessation of breathing
appendiceal	(adj.) pertaining to the appendix, or a dependent part of an attached structure

approximate	(v.) to bring objects together in close proximity
aqueous	(adj.) pertaining to water or watery
arrhythmia	(n.) irregular rhythm or loss of rhythm of the heart
arteriosclerosis	(n.) a condition involving hardening, thickening, and loss of elasticity of the arteries
arthritis	(n.) inflammation of the joints
articulated	(adj.) having joints, or being clearly spoken
aspirate	(v.) to draw out by suction; (n.) the product of aspiration
asthma	(n.) a condition of recurrent attacks of paroxysmal dyspnea with wheezing and bronchial spasms
astringent	(n.) a substance that contracts, toughens, shrinks, whistens or hardens skin or tissue
asymmetrical	(adj.) exhibiting a lack of symmetry or a lack of similar polar or axial proportionment
asymptomatic	(adj.) exhibiting a lack of symptoms or complaints
ataxia	(n.) a lack of muscular coordination
atelectasis	(n.) incomplete expansion or collapse of the lung
atraumatic	(adj.) without evidence of trauma
atrophy	(n.) a degeneration or wasting away of something
auscultation	(n.) the act of listening to sounds in the body, oftentimes with a stethoscope
axilla	(n.) the armpit
Babinski's reflex	flexion inward of the great toe when the sole of the foot is stimulated
bacteriuria	(n.) an excessive amount of bacteria in the urine
basilar	(adj.) pertaining to a base of something, especially the lungs
benign	(adj.) not malignant, progressing or impressive
bilateral	(adj.) pertaining to two sides
biliary	(adj.) pertaining to bile or a bile passageway
bilirubin	(n.) bile pigment
bimanual	(adj.) pertaining to a task accomplished using both hands
biopsy	(n.) excision of a sample of tissue for microscopic evaluation
bradycardia	(n.) a slow heartbeat rate
bronchitis	(n.) inflammation of the bronchi
bronchodilator	(n.) a medicinal device that dilates the bronchi of the lungs
bruit	(n.) an abnormal sound or noise
buccal	(n.) pertaining to the cheek or mouth
bursitis	(n.) inflammation of a bursa, or inflammation of a saclike cavity filled with a viscous fluid where friction would otherwise develop
cachexia	(n.) a condition characterized by malnutrition, ill health, and wasting
cafe au lait	(adj.) [French—literally, coffee with milk] something, especially a skin spot, marked by the color of creamed coffee
calcification	(n.) the process of tissue becoming hardened due to lime salt deposits
calor	(n.) warmth, heat or fever

cannula	(n.) a tubing or sheath
carcinoma	(n.) a cancer or cancerous new growth composed of epithelial cells that tend to metastasize
cardiomyopathy	(n.) disease of the heart muscle
cardiovascular	(adj.) relating to the heart and vessels
caries	(n.) a process that results in the destruction of a tooth, producing a cavity in the tooth
carbuncle	(n.) a small fleshy eminence
catheterization	(n.) passage of a tube through the body for evacuating or injecting fluids into body cavities
caudal	(adj.) pertaining to the tail or end of something
cauterization	(n.) cutting or destroying tissue with an electric, caustic, burning or freezing device
cephalalgia	(n.) headache
cerumen	(n.) ear wax
cervical	(adj.) pertaining to the neck or the cervix
cholelithiasis	(n.) the presence or forming of gallstones
chondromalacia	(n.) softening of joint cartilage, especially of the patella
chronic	(adj.) of long duration or progressing
claudication	(n.) the quality of being limp
clinical	(adj.) pertaining to a clinic or being characterized by observable signs and symptoms
clubbing	(n.) a condition characterized by lateral and longitudinal curvature of the nails of the fingers and toes with soft tissue enlargement
coagulation	(n.) the process of clotting, especially blood
coccyx	(n.) the tailbone, or the lowest section of the spine
congenital	(adj.) present at birth
conjunctivitis	(n.) inflammation of the pink portion of the eyelids
convalescence	(n.) the period of recovery after a disease or an injury
coryza	(n.) a head cold
costal	(adj.) pertaining to the ribs
cranial nerves	the 12 pairs of nerves originating in the brain dealing with the senses and the sensations of the head, face and neck
crepitation	(n.) the sound of rattling or crackling or the grating of bones together
critical	(adj.) urgent or pertaining to a state of crisis or danger
cryocautery	(n.) surgical cutting using coldness
culmen	(n.) the top of the cerebellum
curette	(n.) a spoon-shaped surgical instrument used for removing foreign matter from a cavity
cutaneous	(adj.) pertaining to the skin
cyanosis	(n.) a bluish or purplish discoloration of the skin, due to the deficiency of oxygen
cystitis	(n.) inflammation of the bladder
cystoscope	(n.) an instrument used for internal examination of the ureter and bladder

debridement	(n.) removal of foreign material or dead or damaged tissue from a wound
decubitus	(adj.) pertaining to the state or act of lying down or being in bed; the state of lying down; pertaining to an ulceration; (n.) a bedsore or ulceration due to repetitive lying down or pressure on tissue
deglutition	(n.) the act of swallowing
dehiscence	(n.) bursting open, especially of a wound
dehydration	(n.) a state of excessive loss of body fluid, or removal of water from a substance
delirium	(n.) a mental condition characterized by confusion, excitement, disorientation and hallucinations
dermatitis	(n.) inflammation of the skin with redness, itching, and oftentimes lesions
desiccate	(v.) to make thoroughly dry
diabetes mellitus	a disease in which the patient displays symptoms of excessive urination and signs of elevated sugar in the blood and urine that results from inadequate insulin processing
diagnosis	(n.) the determination of the functional state or a body organ or component; the process of distinguishing one disease from another
dialysis	(n.) the passage of fluid through a membrane, especially diffusing blood through a membrane to remove toxic materials and maintain chemical balance when kidney function is impaired
diaphoresis	(n.) an increase in perspiration
diarrhea	(n.) an abnormal frequency and fluid content of stools
diastolic pressure	the lower reading of the blood pressure; the period of least pressure in the arterial vascular system
differential	(adj.) marked by differences; (n.) the determination of the variety of white blood cells in one microliter of blood
diffuse	(adj.) spreading or scattered; (v.) to spread or scatter
dilate	(v.) to expand or widen
diplopia	(n.) a condition of having double vision
disease	(n.) [literally, not at ease] a condition characterized by signs and symptoms specific to a particular abnormality of the body or mind
disequilibrium	(n.) unequal or uneven balance
distal	(adj.) farthest from the center or middle, especially of the trunk
diuretic	(adj.) characterized by increasing the amount of urine or urination; (n.) a substance that promotes or increases the secretion of urine
diverticulum	(n.) a sac or pouch in the walls of an organ or a canal, especially of the intestines
dorsal	(adj.) pertaining to the back of something
dysplasia	(n.) abnormal development of tissue
dyspnea	(n.) difficulty breathing
dystonia	(n.) prolonged muscle contractions causing body twisting, repetitive movements or abnormal posture
dysuria	(n.) difficult or painful urination
ecchymosis	(n.) a bruise, or the black-and-blue appearance caused by hemorrhaging under the skin

ectopic	(adj.) out of place or malpositioned
eczema	(n.) an inflammatory disease of the skin accompanied by redness, itching and, if more severe, oozing and crusting
edema	(n.) a condition of the tissues characterized by swelling due to the presence of excessive fluid
edentulous	(adj.) without teeth
effusion	(n.) escape of fluid into a body cavity, especially the pleural cavities of the lungs
electrocautery	(n.) surgical cutting with electrical current
electrolytes	(n.) the ionized salts contained in the blood, serums and cells; in hematology, the salts including sodium, potassium, calcium, magnesium and chlorine
emanate	(v.) to give off, radiate or emit
embolus	(n.) a blood clot lodged in a vessel, causing obstruction of blood flow
emesis	(n.) vomiting, regurgitation
endoscopy	(n.) inspection of a body cavity with an endoscope, which is a piece of equipment consisting of a tube and a lighted optical system for viewing through the tube
enuresis	(n.) involuntary urination; bed-wetting
epidermis	(n.) the outermost layer of skin
epistaxis	(n.) a nosebleed
epithelial	(adj.) pertaining to the outer layer of skin or mucosal surfaces
erythema	(n.) redness, especially of the skin
erythrocyte	(n.) a red blood cell
ethanol	(n.) alcohol
etiology	(n.) the study of the factors that cause disease, or the precipitants to a disease process
euphoria	(n.) a state or sense of well being, or the absence of pain or distress
everted	(v.) turned outward, especially the eyelids
exacerbation	(n.) aggravation or increase of symptoms or severity of a disease
excoriation	(n.) abrasion of the outer layer of skin or surface of an organ
exophthalmos	(n.) an abnormal protrusion of the eyeball
expiration	(n.) the act of exhaling; death
exsanguination	(n.) the expression or removal of blood from a body part
extraocular	(adj.) outside the eye, especially the muscles attached to the eye controlling eye movement
extrapyramidal	(adj.) outside the pyramidal tracts of the central nervous system
extremity	(n.) the arm or the leg; the terminal portion of something
extrinsic	(adj.) pertaining to something coming from or without
extubate	(v.) to remove a tube from something
exudate	(n.) material such as fluid, mucus, cells or cellular debris that has escaped from blood vessels and has been deposited in the tissue or tissue surfaces, usually as a result of inflammation
facies	(a.) the face or surface of a structure
familial	(adj.) pertaining to a family or family relationship

fascia	(n.) the muscular membrane that covers, separates and supports muscles
fasciculation	(n.) the formation of nerve or muscle fibers; involuntary contractions or twitching of muscle fibers
fatigue	(n.) a condition of feeling tired or weary
fibrillation	(n.) an abnormal electrical current or contraction, especially of the heart
fimbriated	(adj.) being fringed or having fringed edges
fissure	(n.) a cleft, fold or groove, especially in the cerebral cortex
fistula	(n.) an abnormal passage, usually between two internal organs
flaccid	(adj.) having relaxed or decreased muscle tone
flatulence	(n.) excessive gas in the intestines or stomach
fluctuance	(n.) variation from one course or condition to another
fluoroscopy	(n.) examination of deep structures by means of roentgen rays
foramen	(n.) a passage or opening, a communication between two openings in an organ, or a hole in a bone
frontal	(adj.) pertaining to the front or the forehead bone
fundus	(n.) the body, base or largest part of a hollow organ
gait	(n.) style of walking
gastrointestinal	(adj.) relating to the stomach and intestines
genitourinary	(adj.) relating to the genital areas and urinary tract
geriatrics	(n.) the specialty of medicine in which problems of old age are treated
gingivitis	(n.) inflammation of the gums of the mouth
glaucoma	(n.) a condition in which the lens of the eye is opaque; a disease of the eye in which there is an increase in ocular pressure and hardness of the eye, atrophy of the eye, and eventually blindness
glioma	(n.) a tumor composed of tissue representing neuralgia
glossitis	(n.) inflammation of the tongue
gout	(n.) a condition in which the uric acid level is high and there is a sudden onset of arthritis
gravida	(n.) number of pregnancies
guaiac	(n.) a reagent used in tests for occult blood, especially in the stool
halitosis	(n.) bad breath odor
hematemesis	(n.) vomiting of blood
hematochezia	(n.) red, bloody stools
hematocrit	(n.) the volume of packed red blood cells in a blood sample
hematoma	(n.) a swelling, collection, or mass of blood confined to an organ, tissue or space
hematuria	(n.) blood in the urine
hemiplegia	(n.) a condition in which one side of the body is paralyzed
hemoglobin	(n.) the iron-containing pigment of red blood cells
hemoptysis	(n.) blood in the saliva
hemorrhage	(n.) the escape of blood from the blood vessels, or bleeding
hemostasis	(n.) the cessation of bleeding or circulation

hepatitis	(n.) inflammation of the liver
hepatosplenomegaly	(n.) enlargement of the liver and spleen
hereditary	(adj.) pertaining to a genetic characteristic transferred from parent to child
histologic	(adj.) the branch of pathology in which the minute structure, composition and function of the tissues are studied
homogeneous	(adj.) uniform or consistent in nature, composition or form
hygiene	(n.) the practice or study of good health or a healthy condition
hypertension	(n.) abnormally high blood pressure
hypertrophy	(n.) increase in the size of a structure or an organ not due to tumor
hypnosis	(n.) an artificially induced state of increased amenability to suggestions and commands; an artificially induced state of sleep or semi-consciousness
hypoglycemia	(n.) a condition in which the blood sugar is abnormally low
hypokalemia	(n.) an abnormally low amount of potassium in the blood
hyponatremia	(n.) an abnormally low amount of sodium in the blood
hypoxia	(n.) a state of decreased oxygen; oxygen deficiency
iatrogenic	(adj.) pertaining to a condition occurring as a result of the activity of a physician
icterus	(n.) bile pigmentation of the tissues, membranes or secretions
idiopathic	(adj.) pertaining to something with an unknown cause
immunization	(n.) the process of creating protection from a specific disease, usually accomplished by vaccine
impetigo	(n.) an inflammatory skin disease with isolated pustules
indurated	(adj.) pertaining to something that is hardened
infarction	(n.) formation of a necrotic area of tissue or portion of an organ resulting from cessation of blood supply to that area
infection	(n.) a condition in which the body or a body part is invaded by a disease-causing or harming agent
inferior	(adj.) beneath or under
inflammation	(n.) a nonspecific immune response to body injury, indicated by redness, swelling, heat and pain
inguinal	(adj.) pertaining to the groin region
integumentary	(adj.) pertaining to the skin or covering
interstitial	(adj.) lying or placed between; pertaining to the spaces within tissue or an organ
intravenous	(adj.) pertaining to something contained within or placed into a vein
ipsilateral	(adj.) on the same side or affecting the same side of the body
ischemia	(n.) deficiency of blood to a part of the body
jaundice	(n.) a condition marked by a yellow skin color caused by the deposit of bile pigment into the skin or mucous membranes (also called icterus)
jejunum	(n.) the section of small intestine that extends from the duodenum to the ileum
kyphosis	(n.) abnormally increased convexity in the curvature of the thoracic spine; a hunchback condition

labile	(adj.) unsteady, changing or easily disarranged
labium	(n.) a fleshy border or edge; a lip
laceration	(n.) an irregular tear or cut of the flesh, or a wound
lacrimal	(adj.) pertaining to tears
lamina	(n.) a thin, flat layer of membrane or the flattened side of a vertebra
laparoscopy	(n.) visual exploration of the peritoneal area with a special scope
lateral	(adj.) pertaining to the side of something
lethargy	(n.) a condition or state of sluggishness or severe fatigue
leukocyte	(n.) a white blood cell
lipoma	(n.) a fatty tumor
lumbar	(adj.) pertaining to the low back between the chest and pelvis
lymphadenopathy	(n.) disease of the lymph nodes
macerated	(adj.) softened by having been soaked in water or fluid
macular	(adj.) pertaining to a nonelevated, nondepressed discolored spot on the skin
malaise	(n.) a vague feeling of physical discomfort
malignancy	(n.) a state of getting worse or resisting treatment, especially with cancer
malleolus	(n.) the rounded protrusion on the ankle joint
malleus	(n.) the club-shaped or hammer-shaped auditory bone
mastication	(n.) the process of chewing, the first stage of digestion
medial	(adj.) pertaining to the middle or middle plane
mediastinum	(n.) a wall or cavity separating two portions of an organ; the organs and tissues that are located between the lungs
melena	(n.) blackened stools
Meniere's disease	a disease of the auditory system marked by symptoms of deafness, tinnitus, dizziness, and pressure in the ears
meninges	(n.) the membranes that envelop the brain and spinal cord
menstrual	(adj.) pertaining to menses, the monthly flow of blood from the uterus
metastasis	(n.) the transfer of disease from one organ or part of the body to another organ or part, which is not connected or related to the first organ or part
mnemasthenia	(n.) poor memory not attributable to organic disease
mucosa	(n.) the mucous membrane or moist tissue layer lining a body cavity or hollow organ
musculoskeletal	(adj.) relating to the muscles and skeleton
myalgia	(n.) muscle ache
myelogram	(n.) radiographic examination of the spine after the injection of a special dye
myoma	(n.) a tumor made up of muscular tissue
myopia	(n.) the condition of nearsightedness
myxedema	(n.) a condition occurring as a result of decreased thyroid gland function
narcissism	(n.) extreme self-love

narcotic	(adj.) producing insensibility or stupor; (n.) a class of drugs regulated by law that induces insensibility or stupor
necrosis	(n.) death of an area of tissue or part of an organ surrounded by healthy tissue
neoplasm	(n.) an abnormally rapid growth of tissue showing a lack of structural organization
neuralgia	(n.) a condition characterized by aching or pain in the nerves
neurologic	(n.) relating to the nervous system
neurosis	(n.) a functional disorder of the nervous system; an emotional disorder due to unresolved conflicts, with anxiety being its primary characteristic
nocturia	(n.) increased nighttime urination
normocephalic	(adj.) having a normally shaped head
nystagmus	(n.) a rhythmic involuntary movement of the eyes; the movement may be horizontal, vertical, rotary, or mixed
oblique	(adj.) diagonal or slanting
occipital	(adj.) pertaining to the back portion of the head
oncology	(n.) the study of medicine pertaining to tumors
opaque	(adj.) not transparent, impenetrable by x-rays
ophthalmologic	(adj.) relating to the study of the eyes
organic	(adj.) pertaining to the organs, body structure or carbon-containing substances, usually those substances that support life
organomegaly	(n.) enlargment of the organs, especially the organs of the abdominal region
orthopnea	(n.) difficulty breathing in any position other than upright
orthostatic	(adj.) pertaining to a standing or an erect position
ossification	(n.) the formation or production of bone; the metamorphosis of something into bone
osteomyelitis	(n.) inflammation of the bone marrow
osteoporosis	(n.) a reduction in the amount of bone; atrophy of the skeleton
otitis	(n.) inflammation of the ear
oxytocic	(n.) a substance that stimulates uterine movement
palpate	(v.) to feel or examine by touch
palpitation	(n.) a throbbing or fluttering pulsation or sensation, especially of the heart
papilla	(n.) a small nipple-like elevation or protrusion
papular	(adj.) pertaining to red, elevated areas or lesions on the skin
para	(n.) number of pregnancies ending in births
parenchyma	(n.) the essential parts of an organ concerned with its function
parenteral	(adj.) pertaining to administering a drug through other than the alimentary canal; a drug administered subcutaneously, intramuscularly or intravenously
paresis	(n.) a partial or an incomplete paralysis
parietal	(adj.) pertaining to the walls of a cavity or the formation of walls, especially the sides and roof of the skull
paroxysm	(n.) a sudden recurrence or intensification of symptoms; a spasm or seizure

pathology	(n.) the study of the nature and cause of disease processes
pedal	(adj.) pertaining to the foot
pediatric	(adj.) the specially of medicine in which problems of children are treated
percussion	(n.) evaluation of the body or of a body part by the type of sound obtained when striking it
percutaneous	(adj.) pertaining to being placed or applied through the skin
petechiae	(n., pl.) small, purplish, hemorrhagic skin spots
pharmacological	(adj.) pertaining to the study of drugs and their origin, properties, nature and effects on living organisms
phlebitis	(n.) inflammation of a blood vein
phlegm	(n.) viscous mucus secreted in an abnormally large amount, usually produced by expectoration
pleurisy	(n.) a condition of inflammation of the lung membrane
pneumonia	(n.) an infection of the lungs, marked by inflammation of the lungs with consolidation
polydipsia	(n.) excessive thirst
polyuria	(n.) excessive and frequent urination
posterior	(adj.) pertaining to the back or rear
prognosis	(n.) prediction of the outcome of a disease process and the outlook for recovery
promontory	(n.) a projecting eminence or process
prophylaxis	(n.) a substance that prevents an unwanted effect or disease
proprioceptive	(adj.) pertaining to one's awareness of posture, movement, balance, position, weight and resistance of objects when placed near the body
prosthesis	(n.) an artificial body part or extremity
proteinuria	(n.) an excessive amount of protein in the urine
proximal	(adj.) nearest to the point of attachment or center of the body
pruritus	(n.) severe itching
pseudomotor	(n.) abnormal movements that resemble normal motor movements
psoas	(n.) a muscle in the region of the last thoracic and first lumbar vertebrae
psychosis	(n.) a mental disorder characterized by deranged personality and loss of contact with reality
psychosomatic	(adj.) pertaining to the relationship of body and mind, especially as the mind affects conditions and perceived ailments of the body
ptosis	(n.) drooping of an organ or a body part
pulmonary	(adj.) pertaining to the lungs
purulent	(adj.) pertaining to pus; containing or forming pus
pyelography	(n.) a radiographic study of the renal pelvis and ureter
pyrexia	(n) fever
qualitative	(adj.) pertaining to quality
quantitative	(adj.) pertaining to quantity
radiology	(n.) the study of radioactive substances and using radioactive methods to detect and treat disease
reflux	(n.) a return flow; regurgitation
renal	(adj.) pertaining to the kidney
resuscitation	(n.) revival after the appearance of death
retroverted	(adj.) turned back or tipped

rheumatoid	(adj.) a condition resembling a disorder characterized by inflammation or degeneration of the connective tissues
rhinitis	(n.) inflammation of the mucous membrane of the nose
rhonchi	(n., pl.) rattling or other abnormal lung sounds resembling snoring
roentgen .	(n.) the unit of radiation used in diagnostic imaging; an x-ray
Romberg's sign	an inability to maintain balance when the eyes are shut and the feet are in close proximity to each other
rubor	(n.) redness or discoloration due to inflammation
rumination	(n.) rechewing of food; repetitive meditation
saggital	(adj.) in a forward-to-backward (anteroposterior) position; arrowlike
sarcoma	(n.) a malignant tumor derived from connective tissue
scaphoid	(adj.) boat-shaped; a boat-shaped bone in the hand or foot
sciatica	(n.) severe pain in the back of the thigh, often radiating down the interior leg, correlating to the sciatic nerve of the hip
sclerosis	(n.) hardening
sebaceous	(adj.) pertaining to the oil-secreting glands of the skin
sedentary	(adj.) pertaining to sitting or a lifestyle involving minimal exercise
sepsis	(n.) febrile pathological state due to microorganisms or their poisonous by-products in the blood
sequelae	(n., pl.) any condition(s) resulting from or following a disease
serosanguineous	(adj.) pertaining to something that contains both blood and serum
sialadenitis	(n.) inflammation of the salivary gland
somnolence	(n.) sleepiness; a condition marked by prolonged drowsiness, sometimes resembling a trance, for an extended period of time
spondylitis	(n.) inflammation of the spinal vertebrae
sputum	(n.) mucusy matter ejected from the lungs, bronchi and trachea through the mouth
squamous	(adj.) scaly or platelike
stenosis	(n.) narrowing or constriction of a duct or canal
subcutaneous	(adj.) under the skin
superior	(adj.) above, higher than
supine	(adj.) lying back down, face or front surface upward
syncope	(n.) fainting; a temporary state of lack of consciousness due to cerebral ischemia
systolic pressure	the upper reading of the blood pressure; the maximum pressure of the blood that occurs during ventricular contraction
tachycardia	(n.) a quickened heartbeat rate
tangential	(adj.) pertaining to suddenly changing to another thought or action; something attached only at one point to the side of another thing
therapeutic	(adj.) a substance used in therapy or in treating a disease process
thoracic	(adj.) pertaining to the chest or vertebrae in the thorax area
tic	(n.) an involuntary, repetitive twitching of muscles, often in the face or upper trunk
tinnitus	(n.) a ringing in the ears
toxicity	(n.) the degree of poisonousness

tremor	(n.) involuntary, rhythmic or convulsive quivering or movement of one or more body parts
tumor	(n.) enlargement or swelling due to inflammation; growth of new tissue that forms an abnormal mass
tympanic	(adj.) pertaining to the eardrum; resonant
uncinate	(adj.) hooked or barbed, as in a bone
urticaria	(n.) a vascular skin condition characterized by pale lesions and itching
vertebral	(adj.) pertaining to bones of the spine
vertigo	(n.) an illusion of movement, or the illusion of the movement of objects around a person when movement does not exist; dizziness
vesicular	(adj.) pertaining to small fluid-containing sacs or blisters
viscera	(n.) the internal organs contained within a cavity, especially the abdomen
wheeze	(n.) a whistling or straining sound produced within the lungs due to a narrowed pulmonary passageway
xanthoma	(n.) a papule, nodule or plaque of yellowish color in the skin, due to lipid deposits
xiphoid	(adj.) pertaining to the lowest portion of the sternum or breastbone; sword-shaped
zygoma	(n.) the cheekbone

Appendix B: Common Medical Roots, Prefixes and Suffixes

A comprehensive list of the common English, Greek and Latin prefixes, roots, suffixes and combining forms used in medical terminology, along with their meanings, follows:

a-	not or without (ex.: atypical behavior)
ab-	away from (ex.: abduct a muscle)
abdomin/o	abdomen (ex.: abdominal pain)
-ac	pertaining to (ex.: hemophiliac)
ac-, ad-	to or toward (ex.: accrue time or adduct)
acet/o	vinegar (ex.: acetic acid)
acid/o	sour (ex.: acidulous manner)
acoust/o	hearing (ex.: acoustic qualities)
act/o	do, drive, or act (ex.: active)
actin/o	ray or radius (ex.: actinometer)
acus/o	hearing (ex.: diplacusis)
aden/o	gland (ex.: adenoid)
adip/o	fat (ex.: adipose tissue)
aer/o	air (ex.: aerosol spray)
-agogue	leading or inducing (ex.: pedagogue)
agr/o	catching or seizure (ex.: pellagra)

alb/o	white (ex.: albino)
alg/o	pain (ex.: analgesic)
-algia	pain (ex.: cephalgia)
all-	other, different or atypical (ex.: allergen)
alve/o	trough, channel or cavity (ex.: alveolus)
amb/o	to move about (ex.: ambulate)
amphi-	on both sides or of both kinds (ex.: amphibian)
amyl/o	starch (ex.: amylase)
an-	not or without (ex.: anaerobic)
andr/o	man (ex.: androgynous)
angi/o	blood vessel (ex.: angiogram)
ankyl/o	crooked or looped (ex.: ankylosis)
-ant	capable of performing (ex.: inhalant)
ante-	before (ex.: antepartum)
anti-	against (ex.: antihistamine)
antr/o	cave or cavernous (ex.: antrum of the nose)
ap-	to or toward (ex.: apprehend)
aph/o	touch (ex.: dysaphia)
apo-	away from or detached (ex.: apophysis)
aque/o	water (ex.: aqueous solution)
-ar	related to, being or resembling (ex.: molecular)
arch/o	ruler, primary, old or origin (ex.: archetype)
-arian	believer or advocate (ex.: disciplinarian)
arteri/o	relating to artery or main branch (ex.: arteriosclerosis)
arthr/o	joint (ex.: arthritic)
articul/o	joint (ex.: an articulated bus)
as-, at-	to or toward (ex.: ascend or attest)
-ase	relating to enzyme (ex.: lipase)
astr/o	starlike (ex.: astrocyte)
-ate	specific chemical compound, one acted upon, cause to become, or rank (ex.: distillate)
-athon	contest of endurance (ex.: marathon)
-ation	action or process (ex.: cremation)
-ative	related to or connected with (ex.: authoritative)
audi/o	hearing or sound (ex.: audiometer)
aur/o	relating to the ear (ex.: auricle)
aut-	self or automatic (ex.: autism)
bacill/o	small staff or rod (ex.: diplobacilli)
bacteri/o	small staff or rod (ex.: bacteriophage)
bar-	weight or pressure (ex.: barometric)
bi-	two (ex.: biannual)
bi/o	life (ex.: biochemistry)
bil/o	relating to bile (ex.: biliary tube)
blephar/o	eyelid or cilium (ex.: blepharoplasty)

bol/o	ball (ex.: bolus)
brachi/o	arm (ex.: brachium)
brachy-	short (ex.: brachycephalic)
brady-	slow (ex.: bradyarrhythmia)
bronch/o	windpipe (ex.: bronchitis)
bucc/o	cheek (ex.: buccal mucosa)
cac-	bad (ex.: cachexia)
-caine	synthetic anesthetic (ex.: cocaine)
calc/o	stone, lime, heel (ex.: calcaneus)
calor/o	heat (ex.: calorimeter)
capit/o	head or large (ex.: decapitate)
caps/o	container (ex.: capsule)
carb/o	carbon or charcoal (ex.: carbohydrate)
carcin/o	crab, cancer or tumor (ex.: carcinogen)
cardi/o	heart (ex.: cardiogram)
-cardia	heart action (ex.: tachycardia)
carp/o	wrist (ex.: carpal tunnel syndrome)
cat(a)-	down, negative (ex.: cataract)
caud/o	tail (ex.: the caudal end of the parotid gland)
cav/o	hollow (ex.: concavity)
-cele	tumor, swelling or hernia (ex.: varicocele)
celi/o	belly (ex.: celiocentesis)
cent/o	hundred (ex.: centimeter)
-centesis	puncture (ex.: amniocentesis)
centr/o	central part (ex.: centrifugal force)
cephal/o	head (ex.: encephalopathy)
cer/o	wax (ex.: cerumen)
cerebr/o	brain (ex.: cerebral palsy)
cervic/o	neck or constricted part of an organ (ex.: cervical collar)
chancr/o	cancer or ulceration (ex.: chancre sore)
cheil/o	lip (ex.: cheilosis)
chem/o	chemical (ex.: chemotherapy)
chir/o	hand (ex.: chiropractic)
chlor/o	green or greenish-yellow (ex.: chlorophyll)
chol/o	bile or gall (ex.: cholelithiasis)
chondr/o	cartilage (ex.: chondroma)
chord/o	string or cord (ex.: chordae)
chori/o	protective fetal membrane (ex.: chorionic)
chrom/o	colored or relating to color or chromatin (ex.: chromosome)
chron/o	time (ex.: chronological order)
chy/o	fluid or pour (ex.: ecchymosis)
cid/o	kill (ex.: insecticide)
cili/o	eyelid (ex.: ciliary body)
cine/o	motion picture (ex.: cineangiography)

-cipient	one who receives (ex.: recipient)
circum-	around (ex.: circumference)
cis/o	cut or kill (ex.: incisor)
-cision	surgical cutting (ex.: excision)
clus/o	shut (ex.: occlusion)
co-	with or together (ex.: cohabitate)
-coel(e)	hollow (ex.: blastocoel)
colon/o	relating to the lower intestine (ex.: colonoscopy)
colp/o	hollow or vagina (ex.: colporrhaphy)
com-	with or together (ex.: communal)
con-	with or together (ex.: contraction)
corp/o-	body (ex.: corpuscle)
crani/o	skull (ex.: craniotomy)
cruc/o	cross-shaped (ex.: cruciate)
cry/o	cold (ex.: cryogenesis)
crypt/o	hidden, concealed or buried (ex.: cryptograph)
cult/o	tend or cultivate (ex.: culture media)
cut/o	skin (ex.: cutaneous)
cyan/o	blue (ex.: cyanosis)
cycl/o	circle or cycle (ex.: cyclohexane)
cyst/o	bladder (ex.: cystitis)
cyt/o	cell (ex.: cytology)
-cyte	type of cell (ex.: lymphocyte)
dacry/o	liquid tear (ex.: dacryoblennorrhea)
dactyl/o	finger, toe or digit (ex.: dactylitis)
de-	reverse, down from or reduce (ex.: decompose)
dec-	ten (ex.: decade)
dent/o	tooth (ex.: dentist)
dermat/o	skin (ex.: dermatology)
dextr/o	right or toward the right (ex.: ambidextrous)
di-	double, twice or two (ex.: diurnal)
dia-	through, apart or across (ex.: diameter)
didym/o	twin (ex.: epididymis)
digit/o	finger or toe (ex.: digitation)
dipl/o	double (ex.: diplacusis)
dis-, dys-	opposite, not, apart, away from, bad, or malfunctioning (ex.: disjointed or dysfunction)
disc/o	relating to disk (ex.: discus)
dors/o	back (ex.: dorsolithotomy)
drom/o	running or course (ex.: palindromia)
du(o)-	two or twice (ex.: duipara)
duct/o	path, lead or conduct (ex.: ductitis)
duoden/o	twelve or relating to duodenum (ex.: duodenal ulcer)
dur/o	hard or to last (ex.: induration)

dynam/o	power (ex.: dynamic)
e-	not, missing, away from or out from (ex.: edentulous)
ec-	out of (ex.: eccentric)
ecto-	outside (ex.: ectoplasmic)
-ectomy	surgical removal of (ex.: lobectomy)
ede-	swell (ex.: edema)
electr/o	pertaining to something electrical (ex.: electron)
-emia	condition of the blood (ex.: hyperemia)
end(o)-	inside (ex.: endarteritis)
enter/o	intestine (ex.: dysenteric)
epi-	upon, after or in addition (ex.: epicondylar)
erg/o	work or energy (ex.: ergonomics)
crythr/o	red (ex.: erythrocyte)
esthes/o	perceive or feel (ex.: anesthesia)
eu-	good, normal or wellness (ex.: euphoric)
ex-, exo-	out of, outside, and the end of, not or former (ex.: extremity or exoskeleton)
extra-	outside of or beyond (ex.: extrapyramidal)
faci/o	face (ex.: facial)
fasci/o	band (ex.: fasciitis)
febr/o	fever (ex.: afebrile)
fect/o	make or agent (ex.: infected)
ferr/o, ferrat/o	iron (ex.: ferrous oxide or ferratin)
fibr/o	fiber (ex.: fibrin)
fil/o	thread (ex.: filament)
fissi/o	split (ex.: nuclear fission)
flagell/o	whip (ex.: flagellum)
flav/o	yellow (ex.: riboflavin)
flect/o	bend (ex.: inflection)
flex/o	bend (ex.: flexor tendon)
flu/o, fluor/o	flow (ex.: fluoroscopy)
for/o	opening or door (ex.: perforate)
-form	shape (ex.: cuneiform)
fract/o	break (ex.: fracture)
front/o	forehead or front (ex.: bifrontal headache)
fug/o	drive away or flee (ex.: centrifugal force)
funct/o	perform, serve or function (ex.: dysfunction)
fus/o	pour (ex.: diffuse)
galact/o	milk (ex.: galactorrhea)
gam/o, games/o	marriage (ex.: gamete)
gangli/o	swelling or plexus (ex.: ganglion cyst)
gastr/o	stomach (ex.: gastric acid)
ge/o	earth, ground or soil (ex.: geology)
gelat/o	freeze, congeal or gel (ex.: gelatinous fluid)

gemin/o	twin or double (ex.: bigeminy)
gen/o	become, be produced or originate (ex.: genesis)
gest/o	bear or carry (ex.: gestational period)
gloss/o	tongue (ex.: glossitis)
glott/o	tongue or speak (ex.: epiglottis)
gluc/o, glyc/o	sweet or sugar (ex.: glucose or glyceride)
glutin/o	glue (ex.: agglutinin)
gnath/o	jaw (ex.: retrognathic)
gn/o	to know or recognize (ex.: diagnosis)
gradi/o	step or degree (ex.: gradient)
-gram, -graph	write or record (ex.: electrocardiogram)
granul/o	grain or particle (ex.: agranuloma)
gravid/o	heavy or pregnant (ex.: multigravida)
gynec/o	woman or female (ex.: gynecologist)
gyr/o	ring or circular (ex.: gyroscope)
hect-	hundred (ex.: hectometer)
hem/o, hemat/o	blood (ex.: hematology)
hemi-	half (ex.: hemiplegia)
hepat/o	liver (ex.: hepatitis)
hept-	seven (ex.: heptagon)
heredit/o	heir (ex.: hereditary)
hex-	six (ex.: hexagon)
hist/o	wet or tissue (ex.: histology)
hom-	common or same (ex.: homogenous)
hydr/o	water or wet (ex.: anhydrous)
hyper-	above, beyond or extreme (ex.: hypertension)
hypn/o, hypnot/o	sleep (ex.: hypnosis)
hypo-	under, below or less than normal (ex.: hypodermic)
hyster/o	womb or hysteria (ex.: hysterectomize)
-ia	condition (ex.: hypothermia)
-iac	one who suffers from a condition (ex.: insomniac)
-iasis	state or condition of, especially pathological (ex.: hypochondriasis)
iatr/o	medical or physician (ex.: podiatrist)
il-	not (ex.: illiterate)
ile/o	relating to the ileum or ileus (ex.: ileostomy)
ili/o	relating to the ilium (ex.: sacroiliac)
im-, in-	not (ex.: imperfect)
infra-	beneath (ex.: infraorbital)
insul/o	island or isolate (ex.: insulin)
inter-	between (ex.: interstate)
intra-	within (ex.: intraocular)
ir-	not, in or on (ex.: irradiate)
irid-	rainbow or multicolored (ex.: iridescent)

ischi/o	hip or hunch (ex.: ischial)
-itis	inflammatory condition (ex.: endocarditis)
jac/o	throw (ex.: ejaculation)
-ject	throw (ex.: reject)
jejun/o	hungry or not partaking of food (ex.: jejunostomy)
jug/o	yoke or join (ex.: conjugate)
junct/o	yoke or join (ex.: conjunction)
kary/o	nut, kernel or nucleus (ex.: megakaryocyte)
kerat/o	horn (ex.: keratin)
kilo-	thousand (ex.: kilogram)
labi/o	lip (ex.: labial)
lact/o	milk (ex.: lactation)
lapar/o	flank (ex.: laparoscopy)
laryng/o-	windpipe (ex.: laryngitis)
lat/o	bear or carry (ex.: elation)
later/o	side (ex.: bilateral)
lep/o	take or seize (ex.: epilepsy)
leuk/o	white (ex.: leukocytosis)
lig/o	bind or tie (ex.: ligament)
lingu/o	tongue or speech (ex.: linguistics)
lip/o	fat (ex.: lipids)
-lith	stone formation of (ex.: tonsillolith)
lith/o	stone (ex.: cholelithiasis)
loc/o	place (ex.: locomotion)
log/o	speak, thought or discourse (ex.: dialogue)
-logy	study of (ex.: biology)
lumb/o	loin (ex.: lumbosacral spine)
lymph/o	water or white cell containing plasma (ex.: lymphatic system)
-lysis	breaking down or decomposition (ex.: electrolysis)
lyso/o, lyt/o	loose or dissolve (ex.: lysis or catalytic)
macro-	long or large (ex.: macrophage)
mal-	bad or abnormal (ex.: malnutrition)
malac/o	soft (ex.: chondromalacia)
mamm/o	breast (ex.: mammary glands)
man/o	hand (ex.: bimanual examination)
mandibul/o	chin (ex.: mandibular)
-mania	mental abnormality (ex.: kleptomania)
mast/o	breast (ex.: gynecomastia)
medi(a)-	middle or median (ex.: mediastinum)
mega-	great, large or multiple (ex.: megaphone)
megal/o	great or large (ex.: cardiomegaly)
melan/o	black (ex.: melanoma)
men/o	month (ex.: dysmenorrhea)
mening/o	membrane, especially of the brain and spinal cord (ex.: meningeal)

ment/o	mind (ex.: dementia)
-mer	part (ex.: polymer)
mes/o	middle (ex.: mesoappendix)
meta-	after, beyond or accompanying (ex.: metatarsal)
metr/o	measure (ex.: pelvimetry)
metri/o	womb (ex.: endometriosis)
-metry	measurement of (ex.: optometry)
micro-	short or small (ex.: microscopic)
milli-	thousand or thousandth (ex.: millimeter)
mis/o, mit/o	send (ex.: remission or omitted)
mne/o	memory or remember (ex.: amnesia)
mono-	only or sole (ex.: monologue)
morph/o	shape or form (ex.: morphogenesis)
-mortem	death (ex.: postmortem)
mot/o	move (ex.: vasomotor)
my/o	muscle (ex.: myasthenia gravis)
myc/o	fungus (ex.: streptomycin)
myel/o	marrow (ex.: myelography)
myring/o	membrane (ex.: myringoscopy)
myx/o	mucus (ex.: myxedema)
narc/o	numbness or lethargy (ex.: narcolepsy)
nas/o	nose (ex.: nasopharyngeal)
necr/o	death or corpse (ex.: necrosis)
neo-	young or new (ex.: neonatal)
nephr/o	kidney (ex.: pyelonephritis)
neur/o	nerve (ex.: neurologic)
nod/o	knot (ex.: nodule)
nom/o	law (ex.: nomenclature)
non-	nine (ex.: nonagon)
nutri/o	nourish (ex.: nutrition)
ob-, oc-	against, toward or inverse (ex.: obverse or occlusion)
ocul/o	eye (ex.: intraocular)
(o)dont/o	tooth (ex.: orthodontist)
odyn/o	pain or distress (ex.: gastrodynia)
-oid	form, shape (ex.: ovoid)
ol/o	oil (ex.: cholesterolemia)
olig/o	few or small (ex.: oligodontia)
-oma	tumor (ex.: sarcoma)
ooph/o	egg (ex.: oophorectomy)
ophthalm/o	eye or vision (ex.: ophthalmoscope)
opt/o	see (ex.: optometrist)
or/o	mouth (ex.: transoral)
orbit/o	circle or round (ex.: periorbital)
orchi/o	testicle (ex.: orchitis)

organ/o	implement, instrument or organ (ex.: organomegaly)
ortho-	straight, right, correct or normal (ex.: orthopnea)
-osis	syndrome, especially pathological (ex.: halitosis)
osse/o, ossi/o	bone (ex.: osseous)
oste/o	bone (ex.: osteopathy)
ot/o	ear (ex.: otology)
ov/o	egg (ex.: ovoid)
oxy/o	sharp or relating to oxygen (ex.: oxytocin)
pachy/o	thick or thicken (ex.: pachydermatosis)
par/o	to give birth (ex.: multiparous)
para-	beside or beyond (ex.: parameter)
-partum	birth (ex.: prepartum)
partur/o	bear or give birth (ex.: parturition)
path/o	disease or sickness (ex.: pathogen)
-pathy	disease process (ex.: adenopathy)
ped/o	foot (ex.: pedal edema)
pedi/o	child (ex.: pediatrician)
-pel	drive, pull or send forth (ex.: compel)
pell/o	skin or hide (ex.: pellagra)
-pellent	something that drives, pulls or sends forth (ex.: repellent)
pen/o	need or lack of (ex.: erythrocytopenia)
-pend	hanging down (ex.: append)
pent-	five (ex.: pentameter)
peps/o	digest (ex.: dyspepsia)
per-	through (ex.: perambulate)
peri-	around (ex.: perimeter)
phac/o	lentil or lens (ex.: phacotoxic)
phag/o	eat (ex.: phagocytosis)
pharmac/o	drug (ex.: pharmacology)
pharyng/o	throat (ex.: pharyngitis)
phasi/o	speak (ex.: dysphasia)
-phery	bear or support (ex.: periphery)
-philia, -philic	to like or have an affinity for (ex.: hydrophilia or lymphophilic)
phleb/o	vein (ex.: phlebolith)
phlegm/o	burn or inflame (ex.: phlegmatic)
-phobia, -phobic	fear of or repulsion to (ex.: photophobia or acrophobic)
phon/o	sound (ex.: phonation)
phot/o	light (ex.: photophobia)
phragm/o	fence or wall (ex.: diaphragmatic)
phren/o	mind or midriff (ex.: costophrenic)
phy/o	to beget or bring forth (ex.: osteophyte)
phylact/o	guard (ex.: prophylactic)
physem/o	blow or inflate (ex.: emphysema)
pil/o	hair (ex.: depilatory)

placent/o	cake (ex.: placenta)
-plasm	form or formation (ex.: neoplasm)
plast/o	mold or shape (ex.: myringoplastic)
-plasty	surgical repair (ex.: angioplasty)
plat/o-	broad or flat (ex.: platypus)
pleg/o	strike or paralysis (ex.: paraplegic)
-plegia	paralytic condition (ex.: hemiplegia)
-plete	state of fill (ex.: replete)
pleur/o	rib, side or lateral (ex.: pleural effusion)
plex/o	strike or paralysis (ex.: apoplexy)
plic/o	fold (ex.: duplicate)
pne/o	breathing (ex.: orthopnea)
-pnea	breathing condition, especially pathologic (ex.: dyspnea)
-pneum-	breath or air or relating to lung (ex.: pneumatic pressure)
pod/o	foot (ex.: podiatry)
pol/o	pole or sphere (ex.: polar)
-poly, poly-	much or many (ex.: polymorphic)
pont/o	bridge (ex.: cerebral pontine)
posit/o	put, place or position (ex.: deposit)
post-	after, behind or later than (ex.: post-traumatic)
pre-	prior to, before or in front of (ex.: preauricular)
presby-	old age (ex.: presbycusis)
pro-	earlier than, anterior or favoring (ex.: prolapse)
proct/o	anus (ex.: proctology)
pseud/o	false or spurious (ex.: pseudopregnancy)
psych/o	soul or mind (ex.: psychosomatic)
-ptosis	fall (ex.: hemoptosis)
pub/o	adult or mature (ex.: pubescent)
pulmon/o	lung (ex.: pulmonology)
puls/o	drive (ex.: propulsion)
punct/o	pierce (ex.: puncture)
pur/o	related to pus (ex.: suppurative otitis media)
py/o	related to pus (ex.: pyorrhea)
pyel/o	trough, basin or pelvis (ex.: pyelography)
pyl/o	door or orifice (ex.: pyloric)
pyr/o	fire (ex.: pyromania)
quadr/o	four (ex.: quadriceps)
quint-	five (ex.: quintuplets)
radi/o	ray (ex.: radius)
re-	back or again (ex.: reanastomosis)
ren/o	kidneys (ex.: renogram)
retro-	backward (ex.: retrospective)
rhin/o	nose (ex.: rhinoplasty)
rot/o	wheel (ex.: rotator)

-rrhage	breaking or bursting (ex.: hemorrhage)
-rrhaphy	suture (ex.: herniorrhaphy)
-rrhea	flowing (ex.: diarrhea)
rub/o	red (ex.: bilirubin)
salping/o	tube or trumpetlike (ex.: salpingogram)
sanguin/o	blood (ex.: serosanguineous)
sarc/o	flesh (ex.: sarcoma)
scler/o	hard (ex.: muscular sclerosis)
sclera(t)/o	related to the white of the eye (ex.: scleroderma)
scop/o	look or observe (ex.: endoscope)
-scopy	observatory procedure (ex.: fluoroscopy)
sect/o	cut (ex.: dissection)
semi-	half (ex.: semisoft)
sens/o	perception or feeling (ex.: sensorium)
seps/o, sept/o	rot or decay (ex.: sepsis or antiseptic)
sept-	seven, or fence or wall (ex.: septal)
ser/o	watery substance (ex.: serosangiuneous)
sex-	six (ex.: sextet)
sial/o	saliva (ex.: sialadenitis)
sin/o	hollow or fold (ex.: sinus)
-sis	condition or state (ex.: electrolysis)
sit/o	foot (ex.: parasite)
solu/o	set free or dissolve (ex.: resolution)
-solvent	something that sets free or loosens (ex.: dissolvent)
somat/o	body (ex.: psychosomatic)
spasm/o, spast/o	pull or draw (ex.: spasmodic or spasticity)
spect/o, spectr/o	see or appear (ex.: spectrum)
sperm/o, spermat/o	seed (ex.: spermatozoa)
spers/o	scatter (ex.: disperse)
sphen/o	wedge (ex.: sphenoid)
spher/o	ball (ex.: spherical)
sphygm/o	pulsation (ex.: sphyamomanometer)
spin/o	spine or spindle (ex.: spinous ligaments)
(s)pirat/o, pir/o	breathe (ex.: inspiratory)
splen/o	spleen (ex.: splenectomy)
spor/o	seed (ex.: sporogenesis)
squam/o	scale or scaly (ex.: squamous)
stal/o	send (ex.: peristalsis)
staphyl/o	bunch of grapes, uvula (ex.: staphylococcus)
stas/o, stat/o	make stand or stop (ex.: static)
stear/o	fat (ex.: stearate)
ster/o	solid (ex.: cholesterol)
sthen/o	strength (ex.: myasthenia)
stol/o	send or tension (ex.: diastolic)

stom/o, stomat/o	mouth or orifice (ex.: anastomosis)
-stomy	surgical creation of mouth or orifice (ex.: colostomy)
strept/o	twist (ex.: streptococcus)
-strict	draw tight, compress or cause pain (ex.: constrict)
-stringent	something that draws tight or compresses (ex.: astringent)
stroph/o	twist (ex.: catastrophic)
struct/o	pile up or mount against (ex.: obstructive)
sub-	under or below (ex.: submental)
super-	beyond or extreme (ex.: supersede)
sym-, syn-	with or together (ex.: sympathy)
tachy-	fast or quickened (ex.: tachycardia)
tact/o	touch or feel (ex.: tactile)
-taxia	order or arrangement (ex.: ataxia)
tect/o	cover (ex.: protection)
tegument/o	cover (ex.: integumentary)
tele-	far, at a distance (ex.: telescopic)
tempor/o	time or temple (ex.: temporomandibular)
ten/o, tend/o	stretch (ex.: tendinitis)
test/o	relating to the testicle (ex.: testitis)
tetra-	four (ex.: tetrahedron)
therap/o	treatment (ex.: therapeutic)
therm/o	heat (ex.: thermodynamics)
-thesis	act of putting or placing (ex.: prosthesis)
thi/o	sulfur (ex.: thioglycolate)
thorac/o	chest (ex.: thoracolumbar)
thromb/o	lump or clot (ex.: thrombocytopenia)
thym/o	spirit (ex.: dysthymic)
thyr/o	shield (ex.: thyroid)
toc/o	childbirth (ex.: dystocia)
tom/o	cut (ex.: tomograms)
-tomy	surgical cutting or incision (myringotomy)
ton/o	stretch (ex.: peritoneal)
top/o	place (ex.: topical anesthesia)
tors/o, torsi/o	twist (ex.: torsion)
tox/o	poison (ex.: toxic)
trache/o	windpipe (ex.: tracheostomy)
tract/o	draw or drag (ex.: contraction)
trans-	across, so as to change (ex.: transcend or transcription)
traumat/o	wound (ex.: traumatic)
tri-	three (ex.: triangle)
-trich-	hair (ex.: trichoid)
trip/o	rub (ex.: lithotripsy)
trop/o	turn, change or react (ex.: tropical)
troph/o	nutritive or nourishment (ex.: trophology)

-trophic, -trophy	related to the growth and nourishment of nerves (ex.: muscular dystrophy)
tub/o, tubercul/o	swelling, node or resembling a tube (ex.: tuberculosis)
typ/o	type (ex.: atypia)
typh/o	fog or stupor (ex.: typhoid)
ultra-	beyond or excessively (ex.: ultraviolet)
un-	not (ex.: unrelated)
uni-	one (ex.: unilateral)
ur/o	related to urine (ex.: urogenic)
-uria, -uric	pertaining to a urinary condition (ex.: hematuria)
vacc/o	cow (ex.: vaccination)
vagin/o	sheath or related to the vagina (ex.: invagination)
vas/o	vessel (ex.: vasculature)
vert/o	turn or change (ex.: divert)
vesicl/o, vesicul/o	bladder or sac (ex.: vesicle or vesiculoplasty)
vit/o	life (ex.: revitalize)
vuls/o	pull or twitch (ex.: convulsion)
xanth/o	yellow or blond (ex.: xanthem)
-yl	substance (ex.: vinyl)
zo/o, zool/o	life (ex.: zoology)
zyg/o	yoke or union (ex.: zygote)
-zyme	something that ferments (ex.: enzyme)

Appendix C: Common Medical Abbreviations

Uppercase Abbreviations

Capitalize the following word expressions when they are abbreviated (an asterisk [*] preceding an abbreviation denotes the name should be spelled out, when possible).

AAMA	American Association of Medical Assistants
AAMT	American Association of Medical Transcription
* A/B	acid/base (ratio)
AB	abortio (# of aborted pregnancies); abortion
ABG	arterial blood gas
ACL	anterior cruciate ligament
ADA	American Diabetic Association
AHIMA	American Health Information Management Association
* AKA	above the knee amputation; also known as alcoholic ketoacidosis

* AMA	American Medical Association; Against Medical Advice
ANA	antinuclear antibody
* A&P	anterior and posterior; auscultation and percussion; assessment and plan
* ASA	aspirin
ASAP	as soon as possible
ASCVD	arteriosclerotic cardiovascular disease
* BBB	bundle branch block
* BCP	birth control pills
BE	barium enema
* BKA	below the knee amputation
* BP	blood pressure

* BPD	biparietal diameter; bronchopulmonary dysplasia
BPH	benign prostatic hypertrophy
BSER	brainstem evoked response
BUN	blood urea nitrogen
BUS	Bartholin, urethral and Skene's glands
* CA	carcinoma
CABG	coronary artery bypass graft
CAT	computerized axial tomography
CBC	complete blood count
CEA	carcinoembryonic antigen
CHD	congenital heart disease
CHF	congestive heart failure
CNS	central nervous system
COPD	chronic obstructive pulmonary disease
CPAP	continuous positive airway pressure
CPD	cephalopelvic disproportion
CPR	cardiopulmonary resuscitation
* C&S	culture and sensitivity
CSF	cerebrospinal fluid
CT	computerized tomography
* CVA	cerebrovascular accident; costovertebral angle
D&C	dilatation and curettage
DDD	degenerative disc disease
DES	diethylstilbestrol
DJD	degenerative joint disease
DO	doctor of osteopathy
* DOE	dyspnea on exertion; date of employment
DPT	diphtheria, pertussis and tetanus (immunization)
* DT/DTs	diphtheria/tetanus; delirium tremens
DTR	deep tendon reflex(es)
ECG	electrocardiogram; echocardiogram
* ECT	electroconvulsive therapy
* ED	emergency department
EDC	estimated date of confinement
EEG	electroencephalogram
EG	esophagogastric
EGD	esophagogastroduodenoscopy
EKG	electrocardiogram (also ECG)

EMG	electromyography
ENG	electronystagmography
ENT	ears, nose and throat (otorhinolaryngo-)
EOM(I)	extraocular movements/muscles (intact)
ER	emergency room
ESP	extrasensory perception
ESR	erythrocyte sedimentation rate
* EST	electroshock treatment
ET	endotracheal
* ETOH	ethanol; alcohol
* FB	foreign body
FBS	fasting blood sugar
FSH	follicle stimulating hormone; facioscapulohumeral
* G	gravida (# of pregnancies)
GC	gonococcus
GERD	gastroesophageal reflux disease
GI	gastrointestinal
GP	general practitioner
GU	genitourinary
GYN	gynecology
HCG	human chorionic gonadotropin
HCT	hematocrit
HCTZ	hydrochlorothiazide
HEENT	head, eyes, ears, nose and throat
HGB	hemoglobin
* H&H	hemoglobin and hematocrit
HIV	human immunodeficiency virus
HMO	health maintenance organization
* H&P	History and Physical (Examination)
HPI	history of the present illness
IAC	internal auditory canal
ICU	intensive care unit
* I&D	incision and drainage
IM	intramuscular
* I&O	intake(s) and output(s)
IPPB	intermittent positive pressure breathing
IQ	intelligence quotient

IU	international units
IUD	intrauterine contraceptive device
IV	intravenous
IVP	intravenous pyelogram
JVD	jugular venous distention
KOH	potassium hydroxide
KUB	kidney, ureter and bladder (x-ray)
LLL	left lower lobe (lung)
LLQ	left lower quadrant (abdomen)
LMP	last menstrual period
LS	lumbosacral
L/S	lecithin/sphingomyelin ratio
LUL	left upper lobe
LUQ	left upper quadrant
MCP	metacarpophalangeal (joint)
MI	myocardial infarction; mitral insufficiency
* MMK	Marshall-Marchetti-Krantz (procedure)
MRI	magnetic resonance imaging
MS	multiple sclerosis
NG	nasogastric
* NKA	no known allergies
NPH	Isophane insulin
NSAID	nonsteroidal anti-inflammatory drug
NST	nonstress test
OB	obstetrics
* OBS	organic brain syndrome; observed
OCD	obsessive-compulsive disorder
* O&P	ova and parasites
OR	operating room
* ORIF	open reduction and internal fixation
OTC	over-the-counter (medication)
* P	para (# of live births)
PA	posterior-anterior; physician's assistant
PAC	premature atrial contraction; physician's assistant certified
PAT	paroxysmal atrial tachycardia
* PCN	penicillin
* PCP	primary care physician; phencyclidine ("angel dust")
* PE	pulmonary embolus; peripheral edema; pleural effusion; pharyngoesophageal; physical examination
PEEP	positive end-expiratory pressure
PERRLA	pupils equal, round, and reactive to light and accommodation
PID	pelvic inflammatory disease
PMI	point of maximum impulse
* PND	paroxysmal nocturnal dyspnea
* PROM	premature rupture of membranes; passive range of motion
* PTA	prior to admission
PVC	premature ventricular contraction
QA	quality assurance; question and answer
RBC	red blood count; red blood cell
REM	rapid eye movement
RLL	right lower lobe
RLQ	right lower quadrant
R/O	rule out
ROS	Review of Systems (part of H&P report)
RUL	right upper lobe
RUQ	right upper quadrant
SAB	spontaneous abortion
SCM	sternocleidomastoid
SI	international system (units); sacroiliac
SIDS	sudden infant death syndrome
SMAC	superior mesenteric artery count
* SR	sedimentation rate; sinus rhythm
SSS	sick sinus syndrome
STD	sexually transmitted disease
* T&A	tonsillectomy and adenoidectomy
TAB	therapeutic abortion
TAH-BSO	total abdominal hysterectomy/bilateral salpingo-oophorectomy
TB	tuberculosis
TIA	transient ischemic attack

TM	tympanic membrane	UV	ureterovesical; ultraviolet
TMJ	temporomandibular joint	VBAC	vaginal birth after cesarean
TSH	thyroid stimulating hormone	VD	venereal disease
TURP	transurethral resection of the prostate	VDRL	Venereal Disease Research Laboratories (test)
UA	urinalysis	V/Q	ventilation-perfusion lung scan
UGI	upper gastrointestinal tract series	WBC	white blood count; white blood cell
UPPP	uvulopalatopharyngoplasty	WNL	within normal limits
URI	upper respiratory (tract) infection	* XRT	x-ray therapy (radiotherapy)
UTI	urinary tract infection	* YO	year-old

Lowercase Abbreviations

Use lowercase with the following word expressions when they are abbreviated (abbreviations with asterisk [*] preceding them should be spelled out, when possible).

a.c.	before meals or food	* o.s.	left eye (also o.l.)
* a.d.	right ear	* o.u.	both eyes
a.m.	morning (ante meridiem)	p.c.	after meals
* a.s.	left ear (also a.l.)	p.m.	afternoon (post meridiem)
* a.u.	both ears	p.o.	by mouth (orally)
b.i.d.	twice a day	p.r.n.	as needed
d.	day	q.d.	every day
h.	hour	q.h.	every hour
h.s.	at the hour of sleep	q.i.d.	four times daily
n.p.o.	nothing by mouth	q.o.d.	every other day
* o.d.	right eye	t.i.d.	three times a day

Mixed-Case Abbreviations

Use a combination of uppercase and lowercase with the following abbreviations (abbreviations with asterisks [*] preceding them should be spelled out, when possible).

* Bx	biopsy	MHz/mHz	megahertz
* Cx	cervix; cancel	mmHg	millimeters of mercury
dB	decibel	mRNA	messenger ribonucleic acid
* Dx	diagnosis	* MyG	myasthenia gravis
ECoG	electrocochleogram	pH	potential of hydrogen (hydrogen ion concentration)
* Fx	fracture		
* Hx	history		
Hz	hertz	* Px	prognosis, problem, patient
IgA	immunoglobulin A	Rh	Rhesus factor in blood sampling
IgD	immunoglobulin D		
IgE	immunoglobulin E	* Rx	prescription; pharmacy
IgG	immunoglobulin G	tRNA	transfer ribonucleic acid
IgM	immunoglobulin M	* Tx	tissue; treatment; therapy; transfusion; transcribed
Kcal	kilocalorie		
mEq	milliequivalent		

Appendix D: Greek Alphabet and Common Greek and Latin English Equivalents

Greek Alphabet

Letter Name	Uppercase Letter	Lowercase Letter	Letter Name	Uppercase Letter	Lowercase Letter
alpha	A	α	nu	N	ν
beta	B	β	xi	Ξ	ξ
gamma	Γ	γ	omicron	O	o
delta	Δ	δ	pi	Π	π
epsilon	E	ε	rho	P	ρ
zeta	Z	ζ	sigma	Σ	σ or ς
eta	H	η	tau	T	τ
theta	Θ	θ	upsilon	Υ	υ
iota	I	ι	phi	Φ	φ
kappa	K	κ	chi	X	χ
lambda	Λ	λ	psi	Ψ	ψ
mu	M	μ	omega	Ω	ω

English Medical Terms with Greek/Latin Equivalents (with Some Common Root Forms in Parentheses)

arm:	brachium, brachion	eyeball:	pupula
back:	tergum, dorsum	eyebrow:	supercilium
backbone:	spina	eyelid:	palpebra
backward:	retro	fat:	adeps (adipo-), lipos
belly:	abdomen, venter	fever:	febris
bend:	flexus	finger:	digitus, daktylos (dactylo-)
bile:	chole	flesh:	carnis, sarx
bladder:	vesica	foot:	pedis, pes, pous
blood:	haima (hemo-), sanguis	forearm:	brachius
body:	corpus, soma	forehead:	frons
bone:	os, osteon	gallbladder:	chore
bony:	osseus	gravel/stone:	calculus
brain:	cerebrum, enkephalos (encephalo-)	gum:	gingiva
breast:	mamma, mastos	hair:	capillus, thrix (tricho-)
breath:	halitus	hand:	cheir (chiro-), manus
cartilage:	chondro	head:	caput, kephale (cephalo-)
chest:	thorax	health:	sanitas
chin:	mentum	hear:	audio
cough:	tussio	heart:	cor, kardia (cardio-)
digestive:	pepticus	heat:	calor
disease:	morbus, pathos	heel:	calx, talus
ear:	auris, ous	illness:	morbus
eat:	phagos	intestine:	enteron
egg:	ovum	itching:	pruritus
elbow:	cubitum, ankon	jaw:	maxilla
eye:	oculus, ophthalmos	joint:	artus, arthron
		kidney:	ren, nephros

knee:	genu, gonu	short:	brevis
kneecap:	patella	shoulder:	humerus, omos
knuckle:	condylus	shoulder blade:	scapula
labor:	partus	skin:	cutis, derma
leg:	tibia	skull:	cranium, kranion (cranio-)
liver:	jecur, hepar	sleep:	somnus
long:	longus	spinal:	dorsalis
lung:	pneumon, pulmo	stomach:	gaster
muscle:	mys	swallow:	glutio
nail:	unguis	tail:	cauda
navel:	omphalos, umbilicus	taste:	gustatus
neck:	cervix, collum, trachelos	tear:	lacrima
nerve:	nervus, neuron	teeth/tooth:	dens, dentes, odous
nipple:	papilla	testicle:	orchis
nose:	nasus, rhis	thigh:	femur
nostril:	naris	throat:	fauces, pharynx
pain:	dolor	thumb:	pollex
pregnant:	gravida	tongue:	lingua, glossa
rash:	exanthema	vagina:	kolpos (colpo-)
redness:	rubor	vein:	phleps (phlebo-), vena
rib:	costa	vessel:	vas
ringing:	tinnitus	water:	aqua
rupture:	hernia	womb:	hystera, uterus
saliva:	sputum, sialon	wrist:	carpus, karpos (carpo-)
scaly:	squamosus		

Appendix E: Medical Symbols and Units of Measure

Medical Symbols

Mathematical/Scientific Symbols

Å	angstrom unit	∞	infinity
°	degree	×	multiplied by; times
′	foot; minute; univalent	=	equal to
″	inch; second; bivalent	≠	not equal to
‴	trivalent; 1/12 inch line	≈	approximately equal to
μ	micron	>	greater than
μμ	micromicron	≥	greater than or equal to
mμ	millimicron or micromillimeter	<	less than
π	pi (3.1416 . . . the ratio of circumference of a circle to its diameter)	≤	less than or equal to
		$\sqrt{}$	root or square root
σ	1/1000 of a second	$\sqrt[2]{}$	square root
μg	microgram	$\sqrt[3]{}$	cube root
:	ratio	%	percent
::	equality between ratios	#	number; gauge; weight
∴	therefore	→	causes the following reaction
−	negative (minus)	←	is caused by the previous reaction
+	positive (plus)	Δ	delta; indicates a change
±	plus or minus; positive or negative; not definite (also indicates standard deviation)	↑	increased; elevated
		↓	decreased; depressed
		m-	meta
÷	divided by	o-	ortho
p-	para	/	per; of; fraction
°C	degrees centigrade (Celsius)	χ^2	chi square (test)
°F	degrees Fahrenheit	Ω	ohm
°K	degrees Kelvin	Σ	sum

Prescription Symbols

℞	take		M	mix
p̄	after		O.	pint
ā	before		C.	gallon
c̄	with		gr.	grain
s̄	without		tab.	tablet
S.	write		s̄s̄	one half

Weights and Measures Symbols

$	dollar		", in.	inch
¢	cent		', ft.	foot (=12 inches)
£	British pound		yd.	yard (=3 feet)
ƒ	franc		ac.	acre (=43,560 sq. feet)
℥, oz.	ounce		mi.	mile (=5,280 feet)
#, lb.	pound (=16 oz.)		tn.	ton (=2,000 pounds)

Miscellaneous Medical Symbols

*	birth		1°	primary
†	death		2°	secondary
τ	life or lifetime		3°	tertiary
♂	male		?	question or questionable
♀	female			

Units of Measure

Metric System

Metric Unit	Numerical Equivalent	Example of Use
kilo	1,000	kilogram, kilometer
hecto	100	hectometer
deca	10	decaliter
(unit)	1	gram, meter, liter
deci	0.1	deciliter
centi	0.01	centigram, centimeter
milli	0.001	millimeter, milliliter
micro	10^{-6}	microgram, micrometer
nano	10^{-9}	nanogram, nanometer
pico	10^{-12}	picogram, picoliter

Units of Length with Metric and English Equivalents

	Millimeters (mm)	Centimeters (cm)	Meters (m)	Inches (in.)	Feet (ft.)	Yards (yd.)
1 mm	1	0.1	0.001	0.03937	0.00328	0.0011
1 cm	10	1	0.01	0.3937	0.03281	0.0109
1 m	1,000	100	1	39.37	3.2808	1.0936
1 in.	25.4	2.54	0.0254	1	0.0833	0.0278
1 ft.	304.8	30.48	0.3048	12	1	0.333
1 yd.	914.40	91.44	0.9144	36	3	1

Units of Volume with Metric and English Equivalents

	Milliliters or Cubic Centimeters (ml or cc)	Liters (l or L)	Ounces (oz.)	Pints (pt.)	Quarts (qt.)	Gallons (gl.)
1 ml	1	1,000	0.03381	0.00211	0.00106	0.00424
1 cc	1	1,000	0.03381	0.00211	0.00106	0.00424
1 L	1,000	1	33.81	2.11	1.06	0.424
1 oz.	29.57	0.0296	1	0.0625	0.03125	0.0078
1 pt.	473.166	0.4732	16	1	0.5	0.125
1 qt.	946.332	0.9463	32	2	1	0.25
1 gl.	3785.33	3.785	128	8	4	1

	Milligrams (mg)	Grams (g)	Kilograms (kg)	Ounces (oz.)	Pounds (lb.)
1 mg	1	0.0001	0.0000001	0.000035	0.000002
1 g	1,000	1	0.01	0.0352	0.0022
1 kg	1,000,000	1,000	1	35.27	2.2046
1 oz.	28,350	28.35	0.02835	1	0.0625
1 lb.	453,592	453.6	0.4536	16	1

Appendix F: Reference Values for Common Laboratory Data

Major Categories of Laboratory Data

1. hematology (whole blood, CBC)
2. urine analysis (urine)
3. serology (serum or plasma)
4. toxicology (poisonous or toxic substances)
5. therapeutic drug monitoring

Hematology

(An asterisk [*] denotes that an abbreviation is acceptable for use in sections other than laboratory data; all abbreviations are acceptable for use in laboratory data sections. Normal values are expressed in conventional units.)

Abbrev. Acceptable*	Reference	Reference Abbrev.	Normal Values
	carboxyhemoglobin	carboxy HG	up to 5% of total
	cell counts:		
	—erythrocytes		
	—females		3.5–5.0 million/mm^3
	—males		4.3–5.9 million/mm^3

Abbrev. Acceptable*	Reference	Reference Abbrev.	Normal Values
	—leukocytes		3,200–9,800/mm^3
	differential (diff):		
	+myelocytes	myelos	0
*	+band neutrophils	bands	3–5%
*	+segmented neutrophils	segs	54–62%
*	+lymphocytes	lymphs	25–33%
*	+monocytes	monos	3–7%
	+eosinophils	eos	1–3%
	+basophils	basos	0–0.75%
	—platelets		130,000–400,000/mm^3
	—reticulocytes	retics	10,000–75,000/mm^3
	coagulation tests:		
	—bleeding time (Duke)		1–5 minutes
	—bleeding time (Simplate)		3–9.5 minutes
	—clot lysis time		none in 24 hours
	—coagulation time		5–15 minutes for glass tubes; 19–60 for siliconized tubes
*	—coagulation factors:		
	—factor I/fibrinogen		150–350 mg/dl (deciliter)
	—factor V		70–130%
	—factor VII		60–140%
	—factor VIII C		50–200%
	—factor VIII VW (von Willebrand)	VW	50–150%
	—factor IX		70–130%
	—factor X		70–130%
	—factor XI		70–130%
	—factor XII		70–130%
*	—fibrin split products	fibrin	negative at 1 : 4 dilution
	—fibrinolysis		0
*	—partial thrombo-plastin time	PTT	22–37 seconds
*	—prothrombin time (factor II)	PT	9–12 seconds
	—thrombin time		<17 seconds
	—tourniquet test		up to 10 petechiae
	cold hemolysin test		no hemolysis
*	Coombs' test	Coombs	negative
	corpuscular values of erythrocytes:		
*	—mean corpuscular hemoglobin	MCH	27–33 pg/RBC
*	—mean corpuscular volume	MCV	76–100 μm^3 (cubic micrometers)

Abbrev. Acceptable*	Reference	Reference Abbrev.	Normal Values
*	—mean corpuscular hemo-globin concentration	MCHC	33–37 g/dl
	haptoglobin		40–336 mg/dl
	hematocrit	H, Hct or crit	
	—females		33–43%
	—males		39–49%
	hemoglobin	H, Hgb or Hg	
	—females		11.5–15.5 g/dl
	— males		14–18 g/dl
	hemoglobin A_{1C}	A1C or H_{A1C}	3.8–5.4% of total
	hemoglobin A_2	A2 or H_{A2}	2–3% of total
	hemoglobin F (fetal hemoglobin)	HgF	<2% of total
	hemoglobin, plasma	plasma Hg	up to 5 mg/dl
	methemoglobin	m-Hg	1–130 mg/dl
*	sedimentation rate	sed rate	
	— females		1–30 mm/hr.
	— males		1–20 mm/hr.
	bone marrow differential:		
	—myeloblasts	myelos	0.3–5.0%
	—promyelocytes	promyelos	1–8%
	—neutrophilic myelocytes	neutro myelos	5–19%
	—eosinophilic myelocytes	eo myelos	0.5–3.0%
	—basophilic myelocytes	baso myelos	0.0–0.5%
*	—polymorpho-nuclear neutrophils	polys or polymorphs	7–30%
	—polymorpho-nuclear eosinophils	poly eos	0.5–4.0%
	—polymorpho-nuclear basophils	poly basos	0.0–0.7%
*	—lymphocytes	lymphs	3–17%
	—plasma cells		0–2%
*	—monocytes	monos	0.5–5.0%
	—reticulum cells	retics	0.1–2.0%
	—megakaryocytes		0.3–3.0%
	—pronormoblasts		1–8%
	—normoblasts		7–32%

Urine Analysis

(An asterisk [*] denotes that an abbreviation is acceptable for use in sections other than laboratory data; all abbreviations are acceptable for use in laboratory data sections. Normal values are expressed in conventional units.)

Abbrev. Acceptable*	Reference	Reference Abbrev.	Normal Values
	acetone and acetoacetate		0 or negative
	Addis count:		
	—erythrocytes		up to 130,000/day
	—leukocytes		up to 650,000/day
*	—casts		up to 2,000/day
	albumin		negative
	aldosterone		
	—normal salt diet		8.1–15.5 ng/dl
	—low salt diet		20.8–44.4 ng/dl
	alpha-amino nitrogen		50–200 mg/day
	aminolevulinic acid	λ -aminolevulinic	1–7 mg/day
	ammonia nitrogen		20–70 mEq/day
	amylase		24–76 units/ml
	androsterone		
	—females		0.5–3.0 mg/day
	—males		2.0–5.0 mg/day
	Bence-Jones protein	BJP	0 or negative
	beta-2-microglobulin	β2 μglob.	<140 μg/day
	bilirubin	bili	negative
*	calcium	Ca	< 250 mg/day
	catecholamines:		
	—epinephrine	epi	<20 μg/day
	—norepinephrine	norepi	<100 μg/day
*	chloride	Cl	110–250 mEq/day
*	chorionic gonado-tropin, human	HCG	negative (positivity denotes pregnancy)
*	copper	Cu	<40 μg/day
	cortisol, free		10–110 μg/day
	creatine		
	—females		<80 mg/day (higher during pregnancy and in children)
	— males		<40 mg/day
	creatinine	creat	
	— females		14–22 mg/kg of body weight per day
	— males		20–26 mg/kg of body weight per day
	creatinine clearance		75–125 ml/minute
*	cyclic adenosine monophosphate	cAMP	2.9–5.6 μmol/gram of creatinine

Abbrev. Acceptable*	Reference	Reference Abbrev.	Normal Values
*	cyclic guanine monophosphate	cGMP	0.3–1.8 μmol/gram of creatinine
	cystine/cysteine		10–100 mg/day
	D-Xylose excretion		21–31%
*	dehydroepi-androsterone	DHEA	
	—females		0.2–1.8 mg/day
	—males		0.2–2.0 mg/day
	electrophoresis, protein		negative
	epinephrine	epi	<10 μg/day
	estriol, nonpregnant females		
	—onset of menstruation		4–25 μg/day
	—ovulation peak		28–99 μg/day
	—luteal peak		22–105 μg/day
	—menopausal females		1.4–19.6 μg/day
	estriol, males		5–16 μg/day
	estrone, females		2–25 μg/day
	etiocholanolone		
	—females		0.8–4.0 mg/day
	—males		1.4–5.0 mg/day
*	fluoride	Fl	<1.0 mg/day
	follicle stimulating hormone,	FSH	
*	females		
	—follicular phase		2–15 IU/day
	—midcycle		8–40 IU/day
	—luteal phase		2–10 IU/day
	—menopausal		35–100 IU/day
	males		2–15 IU/day
*	glucose	sugar	<250 mg/day
	hemoglobin and myoglobin		negative
*	homogentisic acid	HGA	0 or negative
*	homovanillic acid	HVA	<8 mg/day
*	5-hydroxy-indoleacetic acid	5-HIAA	2–8 mg/day (women lower than men)
	hydroxyproline		
	— adults 22–65 yrs		6–22 mg/day/square meter
	— adults >65 yrs		5–17 mg/day/m^2
	—infants		55–220 mg/day/m^2
	—children		25–80 mg/day/m^2
	17-hydroxysteroids		2–10 mg/day (women lower than men)
	17-ketosteroids		6–20 mg/day

Abbrev. Acceptable*	Reference	Reference Abbrev.	Normal Values
	lysozyme (murimidase)		<2 μg/ml
*	magnesium	Mg	6.0–8.5 mEq/day
*	mercury	Hb	<30 μg/day
	metanephrines		0–2.0 mg/day
*	lead	Pb	0.08 μg/ml, or 120 μg/day or less
*	nitrogen, amino acid	N	50–200 mg/day
	norepinephrine	norepi	<100 μg/day
*	osmolality	Osm	50–1,200 mOsm/kg of water
	oxalate	OAO	10–40 mg/day
*	phosphate	PO$_4$	depends on diet
*	potential of hydrogen concentration (hydrogen ion concentration)	pH	4.6–8.0, average 6.0
*	phenolsulfon-phthalein excretion	PSP	25% or more in 15 min., 40% or more in 30 min., 55% or more in 2 hours
*	phenylpyravic acid	PPVA	negative
	phosphorus	phos, P	0.9–1.3 g/day
*	porphobilinogen	PBG	0–2.0 mg/day
	porphyrins:		
	—coproporphyrin		45–180 μg/day
	—protoporphyrin		15–50 μg/dl
	—uroporphyrin		5–20 μg/day
*	potassium	K	25–100 mEq/day
	pregnanediol		0.2–1.4 mg/day (increases markedly during luteal phase of menstruation)
	pregnanetriol		0.5–2.0 mg/day
	protein		qualitatively negative; quantitatively <150/day
*	sodium	Na	130–260 mEq/day
*	specific gravity	spec. grav.	1.003–1.030
*	thiamine hydrochloride	vitamin B1	60–500 mg/day
	titratable acidity		20–40 mEq/day
	urate		200–500 mg/day (normal diet)
	urobilinogen		0–4 mg/day, or up to 1.0 Ehrlich units/2 hours
*	vanillylmandelic acid	VMA	up to 9 mg/day
	zinc	Zn	150–1,200 μg/day

Serology (References for blood, plasma and serum)

(An asterisk [*] denotes that an abbreviation is acceptable for use in sections other than laboratory data; all abbreviations are acceptable for use in laboratory data sections. Normal values are expressed in conventional units.) {♣ denotes common SMAC (superior mesenteric artery count) value, ♥ denotes common ABG (arterial blood gas) value, and ♦ denotes liver panel value.}

Abbrev. Acceptable*	Reference	Reference Abbrev.	Normal Values
	acetoacetate		0.3–3.0 mg/dl
	acetone		negative
	acid phosphatase	acid phos.	0–0.8 units/liter
*	adrenocorticotropic hormone, serum	ACTH	20–100 pg/ml (picograms/ milliliter)
♦ ♣	albumin		4–6 g/dl
	aldolase, serum		0–6 units/liter
♦ ♣	alkaline phosphatase	alk. phos.	30–120 units/liter
	alpha-fetoprotein	AFP	0–20 ng/ml (gestation dependent in amniotic fluid)
	aluminum	Al	0–15 µg/liter
♦	ammonia, plasma		10–80 µmol/liter
	amylase, serum		0–130 units/liter
	anion gap		8–16 mEq/l
*	antinuclear antibodies	ANA	negative at 1 : 10 dilution
	ascorbic acid, blood		0.6–2.0 mg/dl
	base excess, blood		0 ± 2 mEq/l
	bicarbonate	bicarb	22–28 mEq/l
	bile acids, serum		0.3–3.3 µg/ml
♦ ♣	bilirubin, serum, total	bili.	0.1–1.0 mg/dl
♦ ♣	bibrubin, serum, direct	bili.	0–0.2 mg/dl
	bromsulphalein	BSP	<5%
♣	calcium, serum	Ca	4.4–5.1 mEq/l
* ♣	carbon dioxide content, serum	CO$_2$	22–28 mEq/l
* ♥	carbon dioxide tension	pCO$_2$	35–45 mm Hg
	carotene, beta, serum		50–250 µg/dl
	ceruloplasmin, serum		20–25 mg/dl
♣	chloride, serum	Cl	95–105 mEq/l
♦ ♣	cholesterol, serum		<200–265 mg/dl (increases with age)
	cholinesterase		620–1,370 units/liter, or 0.5–1.3 pH units
	copper, serum	Cu	70–140 µg/dl
	cortisol, plasma		6–23 µg/dl
	creatine, serum		
	— females		0.35–0.93 mg/dl
	— males		0.17–0.50 mg/dl

Abbrev. Acceptable*	Reference	Reference Abbrev.	Normal Values
*	creatine phosphokinase (also creatine kinase)	CPK, CK	0–150 units/liter (twofold in females)
♣	creatinine, serum	creat	0.6–1.2 mg/dl
*	dehydroepiandrosterone	DHEA	
	—child		0.1–2.9 µg/l
	—pubescent		0.5–9.2 µg/l
	—adolescent		2.5–20.0 µg/l
	—premenopausal female		2.0–15.0 µg/l
	—male		0.8–10.0 µg/l
*	dehydroepiandrosterone sulphate	DHEA-S	
	—newborn		1,670–3,640 ng/ml
	—prepubescent		100–600 ng/ml
	—premenopausal female		820–3,380 ng/ml
	—postmenopausal female		110–610 ng/ml
	—pregnancy, at term		230–1,170 ng/ml
	—males		2,000–3,350 ng/ml
	fatty acids, serum	FA	8–20 mg/dl
	ferritin, serum		18–300 ng/ml
	fibrinogen, serum		<10 mg/ml
	folate, serum		2–10 ng/ml
*	follicle stimulating hormone	FSH	
	—females, regular production		2–15 mu/ml (microunits/milliliter)
	—females, peak production		20–50 mu/ml
	—males		1–10 mu/ml
* ♦	gamma glutamyl-transferase	GGT	0–30 mu/ml
	gastrin, serum		0–180 pg/ml
	glucose (fasting):		
♣	—blood		60–100 mg/dl
♣	—plasma or serum		70–115 mg/dl
	growth hormone, fasting		
	—females		0–10 ng/ml
	—males		0–5 ng/ml
	immunoglobulins, serum:		
*	—IgG	IgG	500–1,200 mg/dl
*	—IgA	IgA	50–350 mg/dl
*	—IgM	IgM	30–230 mg/dl
*	—IgD	IgD	<6 mg/dl
*	—IgE (child)	IgE	0.5–10 units/ml

Abbrev. Acceptable*	Reference	Reference Abbrev.	Normal Values
*	—IgE (adult)	IgE	5–100 units/ml
	insulin, plasma		5–20 mu/ml
*	iodine, serum	I	3.5–8.0 µg/dl
*	iron, serum	Fe	60–180 µg/dl
	iron binding capacity:		
	—total		250–460 µg/dl
	—saturation		20–55%
	lactate, blood		0.6–1.8 mEq/l
* ♣	lactate dehy-drogenase, serum	LDH	50–150 units/liter
	lipase, serum		0–160 units/liter
	lipids, total, plasma		400–850 mg/dl
	lipoproteins		
*	—high density lipoproteins	HDL	30–90 mg/dl (< LDL quantity)
*	—low density lipoproteins	LDL	50–190 mg/dl (> HDL quantity)
*	luteinizing hormone, serum	LH	
	—females		2–20 mu/ml
	—females, peak production		30–140 mu/ml
	—males		3–25 mu/ml
*	magnesium, serum	Mg	1.6–2.24 mEq/l
*	nitrogen, nonprotein serum	N	15–35 mg/dl
*	osmolality, serum	Osm	280–300 mOsm/kg
	oxygen, blood:		
* ♥	—capacity	O_2	16–24 volumes percent
* ♥	—content (arterial)	O_2	15–23 volumes percent
* ♥	—saturation (arterial)	O_2	94–100% of capacity
* ♥	—tension	pO_2	75–100 mm Hg
♣	potassium	K	3.5–5.0 mEq/l
* ♥	potential of hydrogen, arterial, blood	pH	7.35–7.45
	phosphatase, serum:	PO_4	
	—acid		0–0.8 units/l
*	—alkaline	alk. phos.	30–120 units/l (higher in infants and adolescents)
♣	phosphorus	P	2.5–5.0 mg/dl
	potassium, serum	K	3.5–5.0 mEq/l
♣	protein, serum, total		6–8 g/dl
	protein electrophoresis:		
	—albumin		60–65%
	—alpha-1 globulin		1.7–5.0%

Abbrev. Acceptable*	Reference	Reference Abbrev.	Normal Values
	—alpha-2 globulin		6.7–12.5%
	—beta globulin		8.3–16.3%
	—gamma globulin		10.7–20.0%
	pyruvate, plasma		0.30–0.90 mg/dl
♣	sodium, serum	Na	135–147 mEq/l
	sulfates, inorganic, serum	SO₄	0.8–1.2 mg/dl
	syphilis serology:		
*	—rapid plasma reagin	RPR	negative
*	—Venereal Disease Research Laboratory	VDRL	negative
	testosterone, plasma or serum		
	—males		4.0–8.0 ng/ml
	—females		<0.6 ng/ml
	—pregnant		3.8–19.0 ng/ml
	thyroid tests:		
*	—thyroid stimulating hormone	TSH	2–11 μu/ml
*	—thyroid hormone index	THBI	0.83–1.17 of a binding unitless ratio
*	—thyroxine	T4	4.0–11.0 μg/dl
*	—thyroxine binding globulin	TBG	12–28 μg/dl
	—thyroxine, free		0.8–2.8 ng/dl
*	—triiodothyronine	T3	75–220 ng/dl
*	—triiodothyronine uptake	T3 uptake	25–35%
	transaminase, serum:		
* ♦ ♣	—aspartate amino-transferase	SGOT	0–19 mu/ml
* ♦ ♣	—alanine amino-transferase	SGPT	0–35 mu/ml
	transferrin		170–370 mg/dl
♣	triglycerides, serum	TG	<160 mg/dl
	urate, serum (uric acid)		2–7 mg/dl
* ♣	urea nitrogen, blood	BUN	8–18 mg/dl
♣	urea nitrogen, serum	SUN	11–23 mg/dl
	vitamins:		
*	—alpha-tocopherol (plasma or serum)	vitamin E	0.78–1.25 mg/dl
*	—ascorbate (plasma or serum)	vitamin C	0.6–2.0 mg/dl
*	—cholecalciferol (serum)	vitamin D3	24–40 ng/ml

Abbrev. Acceptable*	Reference	Reference Abbrev.	Normal Values
*	—cyanocobalamin (serum)	vitamin B12	20–100 ng/dl
*	—pyridoxal (plasma)	vitamin B6	20–90 ng/ml
*	—retinol (plasma or serum)	vitamin A	10–50 µg/dl
*	—riboflavin (serum)	vitamin B2	2.6–3.7 µg/dl
	zinc	Zn	75–120 µg/dl

Toxicology

(An asterisk [*] denotes that an abbreviation is acceptable for use in sections other than laboratory data; all abbreviations are acceptable for use in laboratory data sections. Normal values are expressed in conventional units.)

Abbrev. Acceptable*	Reference	Reference Abbrev.	Normal Values
	arsenic, blood	As	3.5–7.2 µg/dl
	bromides, serum	Br	toxic levels: >17 mEq/l
*	carbon monoxide, blood	CO	up to 5% saturation (symptoms occur with 20% saturation)
*	ethanol, blood	ETOH	
	—marked intoxication		0.3–0.4%
	—alcoholic stupor		0.4–0.5%
	—coma		>0.5%
*	lead, blood	Pb	0–40 µg/dl

Therapeutic Drug Monitoring

Drug Name	Therapeutic Range	Toxic Levels
antibiotics:		
—amikacin	15–25 µg/ml	>35 µg/ml
—chloramphenicol	10–20 µg/ml	>25 µg/ml
—gentamicin	5–10 µg/ml	>12 µg/ml
—tobramycin	5–10 µg/ml	>12 µg/ml
anticonvulsants:		
—carbamazepine	5–12 µg/ml	>15 µg/ml
—ethosuximide	40–80 µg/ml	>150 µg/ml
—phenobarbital	10–25 µg/ml	varies
—phenytoin	10–20 µg/ml	>20 µg/ml
—primidone	4–12 µg/ml	>15 µg/ml
—valproic acid	50–100 µg/ml	>200 µg/ml
anti-inflammatory agents:		
—acetaminophen	10–20 µg/ml	>250 µg/ml
—salicylate	100–250 µg/ml	>300 µg/ml

Drug Name	Therapeutic Range	Toxic Levels
bronchodilators:		
—theophylline	10–20 µg/ml	>20 µg/ml
cardiovascular drugs:		
—digitoxin	15–25 ng/ml	>25 ng/ml
—digoxin	0.8–2 ng/ml	>2.4 ng/ml
—disopyramide	2–4 µg/ml	>7 µg/ml
—lidocaine	1.5–5 µg/ml	>6 µg/ml
—procainamide	4–10 µg/ml	>16 µg/ml
—propranolol	50–100 ng/ml	varies
—quinidine	2–5 µg/ml	>10 µg/ml
psychopharmacologic drugs:		
—amitriptyline	120–150 ng/ml	>500 ng/ml
—chlordiazepexide	1–3 µg/ml	>5 µg/ml
—desipramine	150–250 ng/ml	>500 ng/ml
—diazepam	0.5–2.5 µg/ml	>5 µg/ml
—imipramine	150–250 ng/ml	>500 ng/ml
—lithium	0.8–1.5 mEq/l	>2.0 mEq/l
—nortriptyline	50–150 ng/ml	>500 ng/ml

Additional Laboratory Data

In addition to the aforementioned values, other laboratory testing of systemic fluids and functioning is often done. This includes reference values for: cerebrospinal fluid, gastric analysis, gastrointestinal absorption tests, feces analysis, semen analysis, pancreatic function tests, liver function tests, kidney function tests, thyroid function tests, endocrine function tests, and immunologic procedures.

Other Laboratory Notes

1. Never begin a sentence with an abbreviation, even in laboratory data.
2. Always use lowercase "p" and uppercase "H" for pH.
3. SMAC values also can be abbreviated SMA or Chem (for Chemistry). SMAC values can be tested either with 4 values (the electrolytes—sodium, potassium, carbon dioxide and chloride), 6 or 7 values (SMAC-6 or SMAC-7, or Chem-6 or Chem-7) or 9, 11, 15, 19 and 22 values.
4. Always use a "0" to hold the place before a decimal (e g., 0.5, not .5).
5. Note that many values increase from threefold to tenfold during pregnancy.

Appendix G: Recommended References and Medical Transcription Resources

Recommended References

(All texts should be the latest edition for maximum value.)

Dictionaries

Dorland's Illustrated Medical Dictionary
Encyclopedia and Dictionary of Medicine, Nursing, and Allied Health
The New Roget's Thesaurus of the English Language in Dictionary Form
Stedman's Medical Dictionary
Taber's Cyclopedic Medical Dictionary
Webster's Collegiate Dictionary
Webster's Third New International Dictionary of the English Language, Unabridged

Word Books

The Medical & Health Sciences Word Book
Medical Phrase Index
The Medical Word Book
Saunders Pharmaceutical Word Book
The Surgical Word Book
A Word Book in Pathology and Laboratory Medicine

Drug Catalogues/Indices

American Drug Index
Physicians' Desk Reference
The Pill Book

Grammar Handbooks

The Little, Brown Handbook
The Merriam-Webster Concise Handbook for Writers
Reference Manual (South-Western)
Webster's College Dictionary
Write Right!

Word Processing References

The ABCs of MS-DOS
The ABCs of WordPerfect
DOS For Dummies
MS Word For Dummies
PCS For Dummies
Using WordPerfect 5.1, Special Edition
Windows For Dummies
WordPerfect for IBM Personal Computers
WordPerfect 6 Made Easy

Other Medical References/Magazines

Accreditation Manual for Hospitals
Contemporary Medical Office Procedures
Current Medical Terminology
DeGowin & DeGowin's Bedside Diagnostic Examination
The DRG ICD-9-CM Code Book
Forrest General Medical Center: Advanced Medical Terminology and Transcription Course
Getting a Job in Health Care
Gray's Anatomy
H&P: A Nonphysician's Guide
Hillcrest Medical Center: Beginning Medical Transcription Course
The IMTA Recorder
The Independent
The Independent Medical Transcriptionist
The Language of Medicine
Manual of Medical Transcription
Medical Abbreviations and Eponyms
Medical Abbreviations: 5500 Conveniences at the Expense of Communications and Safety
Medical Abbreviations Handbook
Medical Office Practice
Medical Terminology Made Easy
Medical Transcription Guide
The Merck Manual
The Modern Medical Office: A Reference Manual
MT Monthly
Physicians' Current Procedural Terminology (CPT 96)
Style Guide for Medical Transcription (AAMT)
Terminology for Allied Health Professionals

Medical Transcription Resources

Associations/Education

American Association for Medical
Transcription (AAMT)
P.O. Box 576187
Modesto, CA 95355
209-551-0883 or 800-982-2182

Health Professions Institute
P.O. Box 801
Modesto, CA 95353
209-551-2112

International Medical Transcription
Association (IMTA)
The Transcription Institute
Box 202
Burien, WA 98168
206-706-2736

Publishing Houses

F. A. Davis Co.
1915 Arch Street
Philadelphia, PA 19103
800-523-4049

Facts and Comparisons
111 West Port Plaza
Suite 423
St. Louis, MO 63146
800-223-0554

Houghton Mifflin Company
2 Park Street & 1 Beacon Street
Boston, MA 02107
800-725-5000

J. B. Lippincott
227 E. Washington Square
Philadelphia, PA 19106
800-638-3030 (order line)

Merriam-Webster, Inc.
47 Federal Street
Springfield, MA 01102
413-734-3134

Physicians' Desk Reference
Division of Medical Economics Data
5 Paragon Drive
Montvale, NJ 07645
800-232-7379

PMIC
625 Plainfield Road
Suite 220
Willowbrook, IL 60521
800-633-7467

Rayve Productions, Inc.
P.O. Box 726
Windsor, CA 95492
800-852-4890

W. B. Saunders Company
Curtis Center—Independence Square West
Philadelphia, PA 19106
215-238-7800

Williams & Wilkins
428 E. Preston Street
Baltimore, MD 21202
800-638-0672

Products and Services

Nationwide (U.S.) Computer Stores

Circuit City
CompUSA
Computer City
Office Depot
Office Max

On-line Services

America Online
800-827-6364

Compuserve
800-524-3388

Delphi
800-544-4004

GEnie
800-638-9636

Prodigy
800-PRODIGY

Other Products

Briggs Corporation (specialty papers)
7300 Westown Parkway
West Des Moines, IA 50266
800-247-2343

Comfort Keyboard (keyboard is broken into
three pieces that can be rotated
in all directions)

Health Care Keyboard Co., Inc.
Menomonee Falls, WI
414-253-4131

DataHand (padded hand rests with finger
wells that operate switches)
Industrial Innovations
Scottsdale, AZ
602-860-8584

Flash Forward (medical transcription
software)
Electronic Ink
P.O. Box 10102
Berkeley, CA 94709-9905
800-653-6826/415-982-5320
                    or
Rayve Productions
P.O. Box 726
Windsor, CA 95492
800-852-4890 (credit card orders)

Intellicat Software (MT software)
Stenoware, Inc.
12337 Jones Road, Suite 200
Houston, TX 77070
800-328-8220

Kinesis Keyboard (traditional alphanumeric
keyboard separated into two pieces)
Kinesis Corporation
Seattle, WA
206-455-9220

Newkey (MT software)
P.O. Box 336
Wayland, MA 01778
508-358-6357

PRD+ MedEasy (MT software)
Productivity Software International
New York, NY
212-818-1144/212-818-1197 (fax)

RayPress Corporation (specialty chart note
paper)
1426 2nd Avenue North
Birmingham, AL 35203
205-254-3731

ShortCut (MT abbreviations software)
Healthcare Technologies, Inc.
610 Village Trace
Bldg. 22
Marietta, GA 30067
404-850-9300/404-955-7555 (fax)

Specialty Business Forms
PO Box 50049
Kalamazoo, MI 49005
800-445-5875

SpeedDemons for MTs (applications video)
IDeal Services
5301 Lindsay Street
Fairfax, VA 22032
703-691-1471

Transcription Services That Utilize Home-Based Transcriptionists

Dictation Plus
800-743-PLUS

Digital Dictation, Inc. (DDI)
800-888-5295

Record Plus
800-944-PLUS

Secrephone/Medifax
800-523-5335

Signal Transcription
800-999-6639

Transcriptionists International
800-466-4326

Transcriptions Limited
800-233-3030

Bibliography

Accreditation Manual for Hospitals. Chicago: Joint Commission on Accreditation of Hospitals, latest edition.

Avila-Weil, Donna, and Mary Glaccum. *The Independent Medical Transcriptionist.* Windsor, Calif.: Rayve Productions, Inc., latest edition.

Billups, Norman F., and Shirley M. Billups. *American Drug Index.* Philadelphia: J. B. Lippincott Co., latest edition.

Chabner, Davi-Ellen. *The Language of Medicine.* Philadelphia: W. B. Saunders Co., latest edition.

Davis, Neil M. *Medical Abbreviations: 5500 Conveniences at the Expense of Communications and Safety.* Huntingdon Valley, Pa.: Neil M. Davis Assoc., latest edition.

DeGowin, Richard L. *DeGowin & DeGowin's Bedside Diagnostic Examination.* New York: Macmillan Publishing Company, latest edition.

Dirckx, John H. *H & P: A Nonphysician's Guide.* Modesto, Calif.: Prima Vera Publications, latest revised edition.

Dorland's Illustrated Medical Dictionary. Philadelphia: W. B. Saunders Co., latest edition.

Fowler, H. Ramsey, and Jane E. Aaron. *The Little, Brown Handbook.* Glenview, Ill: Scott, Foresman and Company, latest edition.

Lewis, Norman, ed. *The New Roget's Thesaurus of the English Language in Dictionary Form.* New York: G. P. Putnam's Sons, latest edition.

Lorenzini, Jean A. *Medical Phrase Index.* Oradell, N.J.: Medical Economics Book Co., latest edition.

Medical Abbreviations Handbook. Oradell, N.J.: Medical Economics Book Co., latest edition.

The Merck Manual. Rahway, N.J.: Merck Sharp & Dohme Research Laboratories, latest edition.

Miller, Alan R. *The ABCs of MS-DOS.* Alameda, Calif.: Sybex, Inc., latest edition.

Miller, Benjamin F., and Claire Brackman Keane. *Encyclopedia and Dictionary of Medicine, Nursing, and Allied Health.* Philadelphia: W. B. Saunders Co., latest edition.

MS-DOS Version 3, Basic Concepts and Features. Vol. 1. St. Joseph, Mich.: Zenith Data Systems Corporation, latest edition.

Novak, Mary Ann, Patricia Ireland, and Frederick J. Frensilli. *Hillcrest Medical Center: Beginning Medical Transcription Course.* Cincinnati: South-Western Publishing Co., latest edition.

Physicians' Desk Reference. Oradell, N.J.: Medical Economics Book Co., latest edition.

Pyle, Vera. *Current Medical Terminology.* Modesto, Calif.: Prima Vera Publications, latest edition.

Roe-Hafer, Ann. *The Medical & Health Sciences Word Book.* Boston: Houghton Mifflin Co., latest edition.

Sloane, Sheila B. *The Medical Word Book.* Philadelphia: W. B. Saunders Co., latest edition.

Sloane, Sheila B., and John L. Dussau. *A Word Book in Pathology and Laboratory Medicine.* Philadelphia: W. B. Saunders Co., latest edition.

Sormunen, Carolee. *Terminology for Allied Health Professionals.* Cincinnati: South-Western Publishing Co., latest edition.

Stedman's Medical Dictionary. Baltimore: The Williams & Wilkins Co., latest edition.

Style Guide for Medical Transcription. Modesto, Calif.: American Association for Medical Transcription, latest edition.

Tessier, Claudia. *The Surgical Word Book.* Philadelphia: W. B. Saunders Co., latest edition.

Thomas, Clayton L., ed. *Taber's Cyclopedic Medical Dictionary.* Philadelphia: F. A. Davis Co., latest edition.

Using WordPerfect 5.1, Special Edition. Carmel, Ill.: Que Corporation, 1989.

Webster's Collegiate Dictionary. Springfield, Mass.: Merriam-Webster, Inc., latest edition.

Webster's Third New International Dictionary of the English Language, Unabridged. Springfield, Mass.: Merriam-Webster, Inc., latest edition.

WordPerfect for IBM Personal Computers. Version 7.1. Orem, Utah: WordPerfect Corporation, latest edition.

Zedlitz, Robert. *Getting a Job in Health Care.* Cincinnati: South-Western Publishing Co., latest edition.

Index